Eat Yourself
Thin
Like I Did!

Quick & Easy
Low Carb Cookbook
by
Nancy Moshier, RN

Acknowledgements

I want to thank the following people for their valuable help in completing this cookbook. First, thanks to my terrific husband Ron for all his critiques of my recipes during the trial-and-error stages of development (he never did turn down a sample!), and for his many, many hours of typing and designing for all these pages.

Thanks to my dear friend Jane Collen for believing in this project and providing moral support and great ideas. Thanks to my parents for believing in my book and me and for joining Ron and my other tasters, Aunt Bev and Uncle Chuck Mueller.

Many thanks to Chris and Robin Ashmore for giving me the idea to create this book in the first place. Thanks also to D.B. Shafer (Shaf) for his help with the computer and a fine job on photography. I would also like to thank Susan Dressel for her expertise with proofing and wording. For the business end of this venture, I've had the good fortune to deal with great people like Jim Meyer, Steve Lange and Dave Swanson at *Gopher State Litho;* Kelly Haskins at *Sitewinder Studios;* Mark Beiter at *Cardservices Int'l;* Nancy Sawyer at *Post Haste*.

We send our special thanks to Harold and Bobbie Gleason for getting us interested in the Atkins Diet several years ago, which started us on this healthy lifestyle and developed our passion for finding ways to make nutritious foods also delicious and satisfying.

Finally, our special thanks to our many friends for ordering the cookbook before we finished it and published it. Now that's FAITH!

Nancy Moshier

Introduction

Before starting, you need to decide which of the low-carb diets suits you best, buy the book, whether it be Dr. Atkins New Diet Revolution, Sugar Busters, Carbohydrate Addicts, etc. then read it thoroughly. I personally used Dr. Atkins New Diet Revolution. After you inform yourself about low-carb diets, you will want to decide what would work best for you and your own circumstances. Although some doctors seem to oppose a high-protein/low-carb diet, many others encourage them. We also know that many nutritionists advocate low-carb diets.

Most importantly, you should check with your own doctor and ask for support and regular checkups to monitor your progress. Although our doctor did not favor our going on this diet, he did agree to support us with checkups and gave us encouraging reports along the way. My husband and I have had great success and even impressed our doctor with our weight loss, reduced cholesterol and overall improved health and energy.

We have tried many other diets over the years and find this one the easiest and most reliable way to lose weight. After losing 74 pounds, my husband has stayed on maintenance phase (about 60-80 grams of carbs a day for him) since April 1999. I have stayed on maintenance (about 40-60 grams of carbs a day for me) since February 2000. We both know we will never gain back the weight we lost. We have made a lifetime commitment and you can too. You can lose the weight you want to lose without ever having to go hungry because of a diet. I hope these recipes help you enjoy gaining a slimmer and healthier life. You have only to make the commitment. With these recipes, you will find it easy to keep that commitment.

Tidbits

When you find yourself too busy to cook daily, make double batches for reheating. Some of the Baked Breakfast Frittatas make a welcome shortcut for those rushed mornings. When friends invite you out for dinner, explain your diet. True friends want you to succeed. Ask if you might bring what you need. If your hosts seem unwilling to cooperate, decline the invitation. When you find that you must attend a function with a set menu that doesn't include foods you can eat, just eat before you go. And when dining out, ask your server for salad or cottage cheese instead of potatoes and bread. Most restaurants accommodate if you explain that you require a low carb diet for health reasons.

I have made the carbohydrate counts for my recipes as accurate as I can, using the data from my research and calculating with standard weights and measurements. I hope you will develop the habit of reading labels and noting carb, protein, fat and fiber counts. For more complete information, see some of the excellent resources available at your favorite bookstore. I use *The Nutribase Guide to Carbohydrates, Calories, and Fat in Your Food,* Avery Publishing; *The Complete Book of Food Counts,* by Corrine T. Netzer; and *Carbohydrates and Fat in Your Food,* by Dr. Art Ulene.

You may or may not have heard of *Xanthan Gum* and *Guar Gum.* These thickeners make a big difference in the recipes. Because it takes very little of them for thickening and stabilizing certain foods, they last a long time and you will find the cost very worthwhile. You can find these products in most health food stores.

I also use Dr. Atkins Bake Mix in many of these recipes because it works well and has a very low carb content. Most health food stores and many supermarkets carry it now. It also lasts quite a while and most recipes call for just a small amount.

Continued on next page.

For cheesecakes, you will find a springform pan most helpful, not only for ease in removing your cake to your server platter, but also for making it sustain the elegant cheesecake shape we have come to associate with this favorite treat. One more suggestion, if you can find them in your area, Daikon radish makes a wonderful substitution for potatoes.

I wish you gratifying success and sincerely hope you find my suggestions and these recipes helpful.

Bon Apetit!

Contents

Appetizers & Snacks 9-20

Beverages 21-24

Breads 25-32

Breakfasts 33-44

Soups 45-50

Salads & Salad Dressings 51-68

Entrees 69-105
   Beef 70-83
   Pork 84-94
   Poultry 95-99
   Fish & Seafood 100-105

Vegetables 106-119

Sauces & Condiments 120-133

Desserts 134-158

Helpful Hints

I would like to help make your diet easier for you by providing the following hints.

Keep on hand:
- *Nancy's Ketchup*
- *Sweet Spicy Mustard Sauce*
- *Nancy's BBQ Sauce*
- *Nancy's Steak Sauce*
- *Salad Dressings*
- *Crushed Pork Rinds* (crushed in food processor and stored in airtight container.)
- *Sugar-free Jell-O®* for quick snacks

Make ahead & freeze:
- *Cooked Italian Sausage* for pizza or frittata.
- *Tomato Paste* - measure 1 tablespoon and 3 tablespoon portions & wrap in plastic wrap, then put in lock-top bag.
- *Lemon, Orange & Lime Zest* – measure & wrap in plastic wrap, label then put in lock-top bag.
- *Appetizers – Ham & Spinach Drops, BBQ Meatballs & Teriyaki Chicken Wings* are just a few recipes that you can freeze ahead and have ready for a quick snack or for unexpected company!
- *Toast & chop nuts*, then freeze in lock-top bags.
- *Taco meat* – measure in recipe amounts and freeze in lock-top bags.

Make sure you always have food available for hunger attacks. Leftover sliced meats, French Deviled Eggs, Beef, Pork or Turkey salad is great on Romaine Leaves. Cubed or sliced cheese is handy for snacks. Pork Rinds and Salsa or Guacamole are also good – just watch the carbs in both of them.

APPETIZERS & SNACKS

BBQ Meatballs 10

Deep Fried Cajun Cauliflower 11

Deli Meat Rolls 12

French Deviled Eggs 13

Guacamole 14

Ham & Spinach Drops 15

Sauerkraut & Ham Balls 16

Rueben Balls 16

Sausage Stuffed Mushroom Caps with Pesto Cream Sauce 17

Savory Stuffed Mushrooms 18

Smoked Sausage Appetizers 19

Teriyaki Chicken Wings 20

BBQ Meatballs

Servings: 32

1 pound extra lean Ground Beef
1/2 cup Pork Rinds, crushed, plain or spicy (optional)
1/2 cup Water
1 large Egg
2 cloves fresh minced Garlic, or equivalent bottled fresh Garlic, minced
1/4 cup Onion, chopped fine
3/4 teaspoon Salt
1/8 teaspoon Black Pepper

BBQ Sauce:
6 ounces Tomato Juice (3/4 cup)
1 Tablespoon Brown Sugar Twin®, sugar substitute
1 1/2 teaspoons Liquid Smoke flavoring

Pre-heat oven to 350°

Mix all ingredients, except BBQ Sauce ingredients, well. Shape into 1 inch balls. Bake @ 350° in 1 layer in a 9"x13" sprayed pan for 30-40 minutes. Mix BBQ Sauce ingredients well. Set aside.

Remove meatballs from oven. Place in deep skillet. Pour BBQ Sauce over and simmer over low heat 30 minutes covered.

32 servings @ less than 1 gram of usable carbs each.

Deep Fried Cajun Cauliflower

Servings: 4

2 cups Cauliflower flowerets, 1" pieces
1 1/2 cups Pork Rinds, crushed fine (0 carbs)
1/4 cup plus 2 Tablespoons Atkins® Bake Mix
3/4 teaspoon Salt
1/2 teaspoon Cajun Seasoning or Seasoned Salt
1 large Egg
1 teaspoon Worcestershire Sauce
1/2 teaspoon bottled fresh minced Garlic, or 1 clove fresh Garlic, minced
Peanut Oil for frying

Wash, dry, and trim cauliflower and set aside. Heat oil in deep fryer or heavy deep saucepan with candy thermometer to 375°. While oil is heating, mix pork rinds, bake mix, salt, and cajun seasoning in a shallow dish. Set aside.

Beat egg, Worcestershire sauce, and garlic in a separate bowl. When oil is ready, dip cauliflowerets, 4 or 5 at a time in egg, draining off excess, then roll in crumb mixture, shaking off excess.

Fry until well browned. Repeat until all cauliflower is used. Keep warm in 325° oven on a paper towel lined pan until all is fried.

4 servings @ 2.5 grams of usable carbs each.

Deli Meat Rolls

Servings: 24

8 ounces Cream Cheese, softened
1/2 large Dill Pickle, chopped fine and drained well
2 Tablespoons Onion, chopped fine
1/2 teaspoon Garlic Powder
8 slices deli Roast Beef, cut in 1/8" thick slices

Beat cream cheese until smooth. Stir in remaining ingredients, except meat. Mix well.

Spread evenly on meat slices, roll up starting on the short side and hold in place with 3 evenly spaced toothpicks.

Slice each roll into 3 pieces. Serve immediately or cover and refrigerate.

Note: You can use any kind of deli meat you like. Just make sure it has 0 carbs.

24 servings @ .5 grams of usable carbs each.

EAT YOURSELF THIN LIKE I DID!

French Deviled Eggs

Servings: 16

8 large Eggs, hard-cooked
3 Tablespoons Mayonnaise (0 carbs)
2 Tablespoons Nancy's Red French Dressing (page 65)
dash Salt

Cut eggs in half, lengthwise. Carefully remove yolks and place them in a small mixing bowl. Mash yolks with a fork, add remaining ingredients and mix well.

Spoon evenly into egg white halves. Refrigerate until ready to serve.

Note: Sprinkle with Paprika for a nice presentation!

16 servings @ .4 grams of usable carbs each.

Guacamole

Servings: 18

1 cup ripe Avocados, mashed (mash with fork, do not purée, should be
    lumpy)
1/2 teaspoon Salt (scant)
1 teaspoon bottled fresh minced Garlic, or equivalent fresh Garlic,
    minced
1 teaspoon fresh Lime Juice (may substitute Lemon Juice)
Jalapeño Pepper, fresh, finely minced, seeded (optional)

Mix all ingredients together in small bowl. Cover with Saran Wrap directly
against guacamole to prevent air from darkening it. Make sure no air pockets
remain.

Refrigerate until serving time.

Note: Use on any of your favorite Mexican dishes, salads, or use as a dip! Only
Saran® Wrap will keep it from darkening. Other wraps are not made from
the same composition.

18 – 1 Tablespoon servings @ .5 grams of usable carbs each.

Ham & Spinach Drops

Servings 18:

1 Tablespoon Butter
1/4 cup Onion, chopped fine
8 ounces Cream Cheese, softened
1 – 10 ounce package frozen Spinach, thawed and drained (squeeze out
    as much liquid as possible)
1 large Egg
1/2 cup Parmesan Cheese, shredded or grated (I use DiGiorno® brand)
1 cup Ham, chopped fine or ground in food processor
1/4 teaspoon Salt
pinch Pepper

Preheat oven to 350°. Place butter and onion in large glass bowl. Cover loosely and microwave 1 minute or sauté in medium saucepan over medium heat until onion is translucent but not browned.

Add cream cheese and mix well. Stir in remaining ingredients until well mixed.

Drop by Tablespoons onto sprayed cookie sheet. Bake about 20 minutes or until set and bottoms are lightly browned.

Serve warm or cold. Refrigerate leftovers.

Note: Also try using mini-muffin cups. They work great! Also great with
    shredded Cheddar Cheese instead of Parmesan Cheese.

18 servings @ .5 grams of usable carbs each.

Sauerkraut & Ham Balls

Servings 8:

2 cups Sauerkraut, drained and squeezed dry. (make sure that
     Sauerkraut is no more than 1 gram of carbs per 1/4 cup)
1 1/2 cups Ham, chopped
4 ounces Swiss Cheese, shredded or cut up
2 ounces Cream Cheese, softened
1 large Egg
1 large Egg White
1/4 cup plus 1 Tablespoon Atkins® Bake Mix
1/4 cup plus 1 Tablespoon plain or spicy Pork Rinds, crushed fine
1/8 teaspoon ground Ginger
Peanut Oil for deep frying

Place sauerkraut, ham, and Swiss cheese in food processor and process until chopped very small. Add cream cheese, whole egg, and pulse until well combined. Shape into 8 balls about 2" in size. Set aside.

Whisk egg white in shallow dish until foamy. Set aside. In another shallow dish mix bake mix, pork rinds, and ginger until evenly blended. Set aside.

Pour peanut oil in deep fryer to line indicated on fryer and heat according to directions.

Note: If you do not have a deep fryer, use a deep, heavy saucepan and a candy thermometer. Heat oil to 375°.

While oil is heating, roll each ball in egg white, shaking off excess, then roll in breading mix, shaking off excess. Let set on waxed paper or plastic wrap while oil is heating.

Gently place in hot oil. Deep fry for 2 1/2 minutes until well browned. Do NOT crowd and make sure oil returns to 375° between additions.

Note: I use Vlasic® or Claussen® Sauerkraut. Also, can be served for a main dish. This is a family favorite at our home!

Variation:
Reuben Balls
Substitute Corned Beef for the Ham and proceed as directed. Serve with Nancy's 1000 Island Dressing (page 68) if desired.

8 servings @ 3 grams of usable carbs each.

Sausage Stuffed Mushroom Caps with Pesto Cream Sauce

Servings: 10

10 large Mushroom Caps (1 1/2" diameter) wiped clean with damp
     paper towel
1   pound roll of Turkey Store® brand hot or mild Italian Sausage
1 - recipe Pesto Cream Sauce (page 129)

Pre-heat oven to 350°

Remove stems from mushrooms and save for another purpose such as omelets or salads.

Place mushrooms cavity side up on a sprayed baking sheet with sides, large enough to accommodate them in a single layer.

Divide sausage into 10 equal pieces and roll into balls. Place 1 sausage ball on each mushroom cap, pressing down slightly.

Bake @ 350° for 45 minutes. Start making Pesto Cream Sauce (page 129) about 20 minutes before mushrooms are done.

Arrange mushrooms on a serving platter, pour Pesto Cream Sauce over and garnish as desired.

Note: Sprinkle with fresh grated Parmesan Cheese if desired. I use DiGiorno®
     Parmesan Cheese and grate it fresh. It's delicious!

10 servings @ 2.9 grams of usable carbs each.

Savory Stuffed Mushrooms

Servings: 9

9 large Mushrooms, for stuffing (wipe clean and remove stems)
2 ounces Sharp Cheddar Cheese, shredded (1/2 cup)
2 Tablespoons Onion, minced
1 teaspoon bottled fresh minced Garlic, or equivalent fresh Garlic, minced
1/2 of a 4.5 ounce can of chopped Ripe Olives, drained

Pre-heat oven to 350°

Lightly salt cavities of mushrooms. Mix remaining ingredients in small mixing bowl. Divide evenly and stuff into mushrooms.

Place in a single layer on a sprayed baking pan with sides. Bake @ 350° for 25 minutes.

Note: You can save the mushroom stems for another use. I often use them in my different egg dishes.

9 servings @ 1.5 grams of usable carbs each.

Smoked Sausage Appetizers

Servings: 16

1 1/2 pounds Smoked Sausage, fully cooked (make sure sausage is no more than 1 gram of carbs per 2 ounces), cut in 1/2" slices and remove casing

1/4 cup Nancy's Ketchup (page 125), or equivalent low carb Ketchup

2 teaspoons bottled fresh minced Garlic, or equivalent fresh Garlic, minced

1 medium Onion, cut in 1" pieces (about 5 ounces)

1/2 medium Red or Green Bell Pepper, cut into 1" pieces

1 Tablespoon Brown Sugar Twin®, sugar substitute

Sauté sausage cuts in a large, heavy skillet over medium heat, stirring frequently for 4-5 minutes or until beginning to brown.

Add onions and peppers and continue to sauté until onions are beginning to look translucent.

Add Nancy's Ketchup, garlic, and Brown Sugar Twin®. Mix well and heat through. Keep warm until serving.

Note: You can use both green and red peppers. Just use 1/4 of each pepper. Not only do they taste great together but they add lots of color to your dish! Also, this has become a huge hit with all my family and friends at parties.

16 servings @ 1.9 grams of usable carbs each.

Teriyaki Chicken Wings

Servings: 9

2 pounds Chicken Wings, disjointed and tips discarded

Teriyaki Sauce:
1/2 cup Kikkoman® Soy Sauce (0 carbs)
4 Tablespoons Nancy's Ketchup (page 125) or equivalent low carb
   Ketchup
4 teaspoons bottled fresh minced Garlic, or equivalent fresh Garlic,
   minced
1/4 cup plus 1 Tablespoon Splenda®, sugar substitute

Pre-heat oven to 400°

Rinse wings and pat dry with paper towels. Place wings on a sprayed baking pan with sides in a single layer.

Bake @ 400° for 1 hour. Make sauce while wings are baking.

Mix all Teriyaki Sauce ingredients together in a medium bowl. After wings have baked 1 hour, remove from oven and brush sauce over wings. Return to oven for 10 minutes. Heat remaining sauce until hot.

Place wings on serving platter or in bowl and pour remaining sauce over wings.

Note: If you like it hot just add a little Tabasco® Sauce to give it that zing!

9 – 2 piece servings @ 1 gram of usable carbs each.

BEVERAGES

Chocolate Shake 22

Strawberry Shake 22

Tutti Frutti Shake 22

Root Beer Float 23

Orange Dream 23

Hot Chocolate 24

Mexican Hot Chocolate 24

Chocolate Shake

Servings: 2

1 cup Heavy Whipping Cream
6 to 8 Ice Cubes, cracked
4 Tablespoons Splenda®, sugar substitute
1 Tablespoon unsweetened Cocoa
1/2 teaspoon Vanilla Extract

Pour cream into blender. With blender running on low, add Splenda®, cocoa, and vanilla extract.

Turn blender to high and add ice cubes one at a time. Stop blender and scrape down sides if necessary.

Continue to blend until thick and creamy and ice cubes are completely crushed.

Note: To lower these carb counts, replace some or all of the Splenda® with liquid Sweet'N Low®.

2 servings @ 6.7 grams of usable carbs each.

Variation 1:
Strawberry Shake
Substitute 1/4 cup sliced Strawberries for the cocoa, reduce Splenda® to 3 Tablespoons and substitute Strawberry Extract for the Vanilla Extract.

2 servings @ 6.4 grams of usable carbs each.

Variation 2:
Tutti Frutti Shake
Omit cocoa and vanilla extract, reduce Splenda® to 3 Tablespoons and add 1/2 teaspoon each Banana Extract, Orange Extract, and Coconut Extract. Add 2 drops red food color (optional).

2 servings @ 5.4 grams of usable carbs each.

Root Beer Float

Servings: 1

1 can sugar-free Root Beer (0 carbs)
1 frozen Whipped Cream Cloud (page 147)

Place whipped cream cloud in 12 ounce glass. Slowly pour sugar-free Root Beer down side of glass.

Add a straw and enjoy!

1 serving @ 1 gram of usable carbs.

Variation:
Orange Dream
Substitute 1 can of sugar-free Orange Soda (0 carbs) for the sugar-free Root Beer. Tastes just like a Dreamsicle®.

1 serving @ 1 gram of usable carbs.

Hot Chocolate

Servings: 2

1 cup Heavy Whipping Cream
1 cup Water
1 Tablespoon unsweetened Cocoa
3 Tablespoons Splenda®, sugar substitute

In a medium saucepan, heat heavy whipping cream and water until hot but not boiling.

Add cocoa and Splenda® and stir until dissolved.

Note: To lower these carb counts, replace some or all of the Splenda® with liquid Sweet'N Low®.

2 servings @ 5.9 grams of usable carbs each.

Variation:
Mexican Hot Chocolate
Add a sprinkling of Ground Cinnamon!

BREADS

Butterscotch Pecan Muffins. 26

Garlic Poppyseed Rolls. 27

Ham & Cheese Breakfast Muffins 28

Hush Puppies 29

Sour Cream Poppyseed Muffins 30

Spice Doughnut Holes 31

Strawberry Walnut Muffins 32

Butterscotch Pecan Muffins

Servings: 12

5 large Eggs, separated
1/2 teaspoon Cream of Tartar
2 Tablespoons Water
1/2 cup Heavy Whipping Cream
3 Tablespoons Butter, melted and cooled
2 teaspoons Vanilla Extract
2 Tablespoons sugar-free Jell-O® instant Butterscotch pudding mix
4 Tablespoons Atkins® Bake Mix
3 Tablespoons Brown Sugar Twin®, sugar substitute
3 Tablespoons Pecans, toasted and chopped fairly small

Pre-heat oven to 350°

Place egg whites and cream of tartar in large mixing bowl and set aside. Place egg yolks, water, heavy whipping cream, butter, and vanilla extract in another mixing bowl. Add pudding mix and whip with a wire whisk until fairly smooth. Add remaining ingredients (except egg whites) and whisk until well combined. Set aside.

Whip egg whites and cream of tartar with an electric mixer until stiff but not dry. Fold egg whites gently into yolk mixture until mostly blended. Use a gentle touch and DO NOT OVERMIX or egg whites will deflate. You will notice spots of white here and there and that's OK.

Spoon into 12 medium, well-buttered, non-stick muffin cups.

Bake @ 350° for 16-18 minutes. Cool 10 minutes in muffin tins before removing. They will fall some. This is the nature of these muffins.

Note: Best when refrigerated and served cold. Great with Vanilla Butter or Maple Butter (page 128).

12 servings @ 2 grams of usable carbs each.

Garlic Poppyseed Rolls
Servings: 6

3 large Eggs, separated
1/2 teaspoon Cream of Tartar
2 Tablespoons Butter
1/3 cup Heavy Whipping Cream
2 teaspoons Splenda®, sugar substitute
1/4 teaspoon Salt
1/2 teaspoon Baking Powder
1 1/2 teaspoons bottled fresh minced Garlic or 3 cloves fresh Garlic, minced
1 1/2 teaspoons Poppyseed
1/2 cup Atkins® Bake Mix

Pre-heat oven to 350°

Place egg whites and cream of tartar in large mixing bowl and set aside. Melt butter in a medium microwave safe bowl for 15-20 seconds on high. Add remaining ingredients to melted butter, except egg whites, then whisk until combined. Set aside.

Whip egg whites and cream of tartar with an electric mixer until stiff but not dry. Gently fold in yolk mixture. DO NOT OVERMIX. Spoon evenly into 6 medium, well buttered non-stick muffin pans. Muffin cups will be full.

Bake @ 350° for about 25 minutes or until browned. Cool in pans on a rack. They will fall, this is the nature of these rolls.

6 servings @ .9 grams of usable carbs each.

Ham & Cheese Breakfast Muffins

Servings: 16

6 large Eggs, separated
1 teaspoon Cream of Tartar
1/2 cup Cottage Cheese
1/4 cup Atkins® Bake Mix
1 teaspoon Salt
2 Tablespoons Green Onion, minced
2 Tablespoons Butter, melted
1 teaspoon Splenda®, sugar substitute
2 cups Ham, chopped (0 carbs)
1 cup Cheddar Cheese, cubed
1/4 cup Heavy Whipping Cream

Pre-heat oven to 350°

Place egg whites and cream of tartar in a large mixing bowl and then set aside.

Place egg yolks in a medium bowl. Add remaining ingredients, except egg whites, in order given, mixing after each addition.

Whip egg whites and cream of tartar with electric mixer until stiff but not dry. Gently fold in egg yolk mixture. Divide evenly into 16 medium, well buttered non-stick muffin pans.

Bake @ 350° for 30-35 minutes.

Note: You can make this recipe extra easy by buying the ham & cheese already cubed.

16 muffins @ .9 grams of usable carbs each.

Hush Puppies

Servings: 16

2 large Eggs, separated
1/4 teaspoon Cream of Tartar
4 Tablespoons Green Onion, include tops, chopped fine
1 teaspoon bottled fresh minced Garlic, or equivalent fresh Garlic, minced
1/4 cup Heavy Whipping Cream
1/4 cup Water
1 teaspoon Splenda®, sugar substitute
1/2 teaspoon Salt
2/3 cup Pork Rinds, crushed
1/2 cup Atkins® Bake Mix
Peanut Oil for frying (Pre-heat oil in deep fryer or use a heavy, deep saucepan and a candy thermometer)

Heat peanut oil to 375°

Place egg whites and cream of tartar in a medium mixing bowl and set aside. Mix remaining ingredients, except pork rinds and egg whites, in a small mixing bowl and beat well. Set aside.

Whip egg whites and cream of tartar with an electric mixer until stiff but not dry. Stir egg yolk mixture into egg whites. Add pork rinds and beat until combined.

Drop mixture from a teaspoon into hot oil. Fry about 3 minutes or until golden brown, turn once. Remove and drain on paper towels. Keep warm.

Note: If you like things spicy try a spicy brand of Pork Rinds along with some minced fresh Jalapeño pepper!

16 servings @ .7 grams of usable carbs each.

Sour Cream Poppyseed Muffins

Servings: 12

5 large Eggs, separated
1/2 teaspoon Cream of Tartar
1/4 cup Heavy Whipping Cream
1/4 cup Sour Cream
3 Tablespoons Butter, melted
1 Tablespoon sugar-free Jell-O® instant Vanilla pudding mix
1/4 cup Atkins® Bake Mix
1/4 cup Splenda®, sugar substitute
1/8 teaspoon Salt
2 teaspoons Lemon Zest, grated, only the yellow peel, not the bitter
    white pith (do not use bottled dehydrated lemon zest)
1 teaspoon Poppyseed

Pre-heat oven to 350°

Place egg whites and cream of tartar in a large mixing bowl and set aside. Place egg yolks in another large mixing bowl, add heavy whipping cream and sour cream and whisk until combined. Add remaining ingredients, except egg whites, in order given and whisk well. Set aside.

Whip egg whites and cream of tartar with electric mixer until stiff but not dry. Fold egg whites gently into yolk mixture. DO NOT OVERMIX, some white streaks are alright.

Spoon into 12 medium, well-buttered non-stick muffin cups.

Bake @ 350° for 20-25 minutes. Cool in pans for 10 minutes before removing. They will fall, this is the nature of these muffins.

Note: Best when refrigerated and served cold.

12 servings @ 1.6 grams of usable carbs each.

Spice Doughnut Holes

Servings: 20

2 large Eggs, separated
1/4 teaspoon Cream of Tartar
1/4 cup plus 2 Tablespoons Heavy Whipping Cream
1/4 cup Water
5 Tablespoons Splenda®, sugar substitute
1/4 teaspoon Salt
1 teaspoon Ground Cinnamon
1/4 teaspoon Ground Nutmeg
1/4 teaspoon Ground Ginger
1/2 teaspoon Vanilla Extract
1/2 cup Atkins® Bake Mix
2/3 cup plain Pork Rinds, crushed fine
Peanut Oil for frying

Pre-heat oil to 375° in deep fryer or use a heavy, deep saucepan and a candy thermometer.

Place egg whites and cream of tartar in large mixing bowl and set aside. Place egg yolks in another large mixing bowl and add remaining ingredients, except pork rinds and egg whites, and whisk together well.

Whip egg whites and cream of tartar with an electric mixer until stiff but not dry. Stir in egg yolk mixture. Add pork rinds and whip just until combined.

Drop by teaspoons into hot oil, frying 4 at a time until golden brown, turning only once. Drain on paper towel.

Serve warm or at room temperature.

20 servings @ .6 grams of usable carbs each.

Strawberry Walnut Muffins

Servings: 12

5 large Eggs, separated
1/2 teaspoon Cream of Tartar
1/2 cup Heavy Whipping Cream
2 Tablespoons boiling Water
1 teaspoon sugar-free Strawberry Jell-O®,
3 Tablespoons Butter
1/4 cup Atkins® Bake Mix
6 Tablespoons Splenda®, sugar substitute, divided
3 Tablespoons Walnuts, toasted and chopped small
1 teaspoon Vanilla Extract
1 cup Strawberries, chopped

Pre-heat oven to 350°

Place egg whites and cream of tartar in a large mixing bowl and set aside. Place egg yolks in another large bowl and set aside. Mix 2 Tablespoons of Splenda® into strawberries and set aside.

Stir Jell-O® into boiling water until dissolved, then stir butter into Jell-O® to melt. Add heavy whipping cream, mix well and stir into egg yolks. Add remaining ingredients, including remaining 4 Tablespoons Splenda®, except egg whites and strawberries, and whisk until well blended.

Gently stir in strawberries. Whip egg whites with electric mixer until stiff but not dry. Gently fold strawberry mixture into egg whites. DO NOT OVERMIX.

Gently spoon into 12 medium, well buttered non-stick muffin cups. Cups will be full.

Bake @ 350° for about 19-22 minutes. Cool in pan on a rack. They will fall, this is the nature of these muffins.

Note: Best when refrigerated and served cold. These are very moist and
wonderful with Nancy's Strawberry Spread on (page 128).

12 servings @ 1.3 grams of usable carbs each plain.

12 servings @ 2.4 grams of usable carbs each with Strawberry Spread.

BREAKFASTS

Cauliflower & Ham Quiche. 34

Crustless Asparagus & Ham Quiche 35

Ham Hash & Eggs 36

Italian Frittata 37

Pancakes With Maple Syrup 38

Pork Carnitas Frittata 39

Puffy Baked Eggs. 40

Quick & Easy Tex-Mex Eggs 41

Salsa Scramble 42

Swiss Eggs & Sausage 43

Taco Omelets. 44

Cauliflower & Ham Quiche

Servings: 6

2 cups Cauliflower flowerets, 1" pieces
8 large Eggs
1 cup Heavy Whipping Cream
2 cups Ham cubes (0 carbs)
1/4 cup green Onions, sliced
1 1/2 cups Cheddar Cheese, shredded
1 cup Swiss Cheese, shredded or cubed
1/2 teaspoon Salt
dash Pepper

Pre-heat oven to 350°

Cook flowerets in boiling water until barely tender. Drain and rinse with cold water to stop cooking process. Drain and set aside.

Whisk eggs and heavy whipping cream in a large bowl. Add remaining ingredients, including cauliflower and mix well. Pour into a 9" sprayed deep dish pie pan or equivalent baking pan.

Bake @ 350° for 45-50 minutes or until just set. Let set at room temperature 5 minutes before cutting.

Note: You don t have to be a big fan of Cauliflower to love this breakfast delight. It's delicious and reheats well in the microwave.

6 servings @ 2.8 grams of usable carbs each.

Crustless Asparagus & Ham Quiche

Servings: 6

2 Tablespoons Butter
3/4 cup fresh Asparagus, tough ends snapped off, cut in 1" diagonal
    pieces
2 Tablespoons Onion, chopped
3/4 cup Ham, chopped (0 carbs)
8 large Eggs
1/2 cup Heavy Whipping Cream
1/4 cup Water
1 teaspoon Salt
1/2 teaspoon dry Mustard
1 cup Swiss Cheese, shredded

Pre-heat oven to 325°

Melt butter in 10" skillet over medium-low heat. Add asparagus and sauté for
3-4 minutes stirring frequently. Add onion and ham and continue to cook for
another 2 minutes or until onion is soft.

Spoon into a sprayed 9" deep dish pie pan and set aside.

In a medium bowl whisk remaining ingredients, except Swiss cheese, together
until light and fluffy. Stir in cheese. Pour over asparagus mixture in pie pan.

Bake @ 325° for 40-45 minutes or until set.

6 servings @ 1.6 grams of usable carbs each.

Ham Hash & Eggs

Servings: 4

1 Tablespoon Cooking Oil
1 Tablespoon Butter
1/2 cup Daikon Radish or Turnips, peeled and shredded
2 cups Ham, chopped small (0 carbs)
1/4 cup Onion, chopped
4 large Eggs
Salt and Pepper to taste

Heat a heavy, medium skillet on medium heat for 2 minutes. Add oil and butter, continue to heat until foaming subsides.

Add daikon radish, cook and stir until radish is browned. Add ham and onion and fry until onion is translucent, about 2-3 minutes, stirring frequently.

Spread mixture evenly in pan and make 4 rounded indentations with a large spoon. Slip 1 egg into each indentation. Cover and cook until eggs are desired doneness. Add salt and pepper to taste. Serve immediately.

Note: Daikon Radish makes a great potato substitute and can be found at some grocery stores in the produce section. It is a large, long, white radish and looks like a huge Parsnip. Very mild flavored.

4 servings @ 1.2 grams of usable carbs each with Daikon Radish.

4 servings @ 1.7 grams of usable carbs each with Turnips.

Italian Frittata

Servings: 8

2 Tablespoons Olive Oil
1/2 cup Onion, chopped
1/2 cup fresh Tomatoes, seeded and coarsely chopped
2 teaspoons bottled fresh minced Garlic or equivalent fresh Garlic, minced
2 Tablespoons Butter
10 large Eggs
1/2 cup Water
3/4 teaspoon Salt
4 ounces Italian Sausage, cooked and crumbled, or more if desired (0 carbs)
2 Tablespoons ripe Olives, sliced or chopped
1/2 cup Cheddar Cheese, shredded
3/4 cup Parmesan Cheese, shredded or grated (I use DiGiorno® brand)
1 teaspoon dried Oregano leaves

Pre-heat oven to 325°

In a large, heavy, deep oven-proof skillet with lid, sauté onions in oil over medium heat for 1 minute. Add tomatoes and garlic and continue to sauté just until onions are translucent. Remove from skillet and set aside.

Wash and dry skillet. Melt butter in skillet over low-heat, swish butter to cover bottom of pan. Meanwhile, in medium bowl whisk eggs, salt, and water until fluffy. Pour into skillet and cover.

When egg mixture on bottom starts to thicken, lift with spatula and let uncooked portion run underneath. When mixture is thickening, top with sausage, ripe olives, tomato mixture, cheddar cheese, then parmesan cheese, and sprinkle with oregano leaves. Cover and slide into oven to finish, about 13-15 minutes or until set. Let stand 5 minutes before cutting.

Note: I cook and crumble a lot of Italian Sausage at one time. Measure and freeze it and when ready to use, it thaws quickly in the microwave.

8 servings @ 2.3 grams of usable carbs each.

Pancakes with Maple Syrup

Servings: 14

3/4 cup Atkins® Bake Mix
1/8 teaspoon Salt
1 teaspoon Ground Cinnamon
2 Tablespoons Splenda®, sugar substitute
1 cup Water
6 Tablespoons Heavy Whipping Cream
3 Tablespoons Cooking Oil
3 large Egg Whites
1 teaspoon Vanilla Extract

Maple Syrup:
1/4 cup Brown Sugar Twin®, sugar substitute
1/2 teaspoon Xanthan Gum
1 cup Water
2 teaspoons Maple flavoring
1 teaspoon Vanilla Extract
1/4 teaspoon liquid Sweet'N Low®, sugar substitute

Whisk dry ingredients together in medium mixing bowl. Mix water, heavy whipping cream, egg whites, and vanilla extract in 2 cup glass measuring cup or small bowl.

Whisk wet ingredients into dry ingredients until fairly smooth. Pre-heat griddle on medium heat. Ladle onto lightly greased hot griddle or skillet into 4" pancakes. Cook until edges are dry and many bubbles appear. Turn and cook until browned on other side.

Maple Syrup:
Mix Brown Sugar Twin® and Xanthan Gum in small sauce pan. Whisk in remaining ingredients and cook over medium heat. Continue whisking until hot and thickened.

Approximately 1 cup of Maple Syrup @ 5.5 grams of carbs total.

14 servings @ .8 grams of usable carbs each without maple syrup.

14 servings @ 1.2 grams of usable carbs each with maple syrup.

Pork Carnitas Frittata

Servings: 6

3 Tablespoons Butter, divided
1 1/2 cups Pork Roast or Chops, cooked, (leftovers work great) sliced
    thin into 1" x 1/2" strips
4 Tablespoons Onion, chopped, divided
1 teaspoon bottled fresh minced Garlic or 2 cloves fresh Garlic, minced
2 teaspoons fresh Lime Juice
12 large Eggs
3/4 cup Water
1 1/2 teaspoons Salt
1/2 cup shredded Cheddar Cheese
1/4 cup fresh Cilantro Leaves, chopped
1/3 cup fresh Tomatoes, seeded and chopped

Pre-heat oven to 350°

In a medium skillet, sauté pork, 3 Tablespoons onions, and garlic in 2 Tablespoons butter over low heat. Sauté until onion is soft, about 3-4 minutes. Add lime juice, remove from heat and set aside.

Melt remaining 1 Tablespoon butter in a large, non-stick oven-proof skillet over medium heat. While butter is melting whisk eggs, water, and salt together in large bowl until light and fluffy. When butter is bubbly, pour 1/2 of egg mixture into skillet. Cover and cook until eggs are set on bottom, may still be runny on top.

Sprinkle pork mixture evenly over eggs. Carefully pour remaining eggs over pork, cover, and place in oven about 12-15 minutes or until eggs are barely set. Remove from oven, sprinkle with cheese and return to oven until cheese is melted, approximately 7-10 minutes.

Remove from oven and sprinkle evenly with cilantro leaves, tomato, and remaining 1 Tablespoon onion. Let set 5 minutes before cutting.

Note: Serve with Salsa if desired but be sure to count the extra carbs.

6 servings @ 2.3 grams of usable carbs each.

Puffy Baked Eggs

Servings: 12

2 Tablespoons Butter
18 large Eggs
1 cup Sour Cream
1/2 cup Heavy Whipping Cream
1/2 cup Water
2 teaspoons Salt
1/4 cup Green Onion, sliced with tops
3 Tablespoons Hormel® Real Bacon Bits (in a jar) or chopped cooked
    Bacon
1 cup Cheddar Cheese, shredded (1/2 of an 8 ounce package)

Pre-heat oven to 325°

Melt butter in 9"x13" baking pan in oven for about 5 minutes. Whisk all ingredients well except green onion, bacon bits, and cheese. Add green onion, mix well, and pour into prepared pan.

Bake about 35 minutes or until eggs are set. Sprinkle with bacon bits then cheese. Return to oven until cheese is melted, about 5 minutes.

Note: Store in refrigerator. Keeps well for at least 5 days. Reheats well in microwave on medium. If your microwave only has high and defrost, use defrost until hot. High will make the cheese hard and rubbery. Makes for a quick breakfast to have on hand for those frantic mornings.

12 servings @ 1.6 grams of usable carbs each.

Quick & Easy Tex-Mex Eggs

Servings: 2

1 Tablespoon Butter
1 cup Taco Meat (page 83)
6 large Eggs
1/2 cup canned Tomatoes with Green Chiles
3/4 cup Cheddar Cheese, shredded
Salt and Pepper to taste

Heat 10" heavy, non-stick skillet over medium-low heat for 3 minutes. Add butter and swish to cover bottom of pan. Spread taco meat evenly in skillet and cover for 1-2 minutes to heat through.

Meanwhile, break eggs carefully in small bowl. Gently pour over taco meat taking care not to break yolks. Salt and pepper to taste.

Carefully spoon tomatoes with green chiles over eggs. Cover and cook until eggs are almost done to your liking. Remove cover, sprinkle with cheese and replace cover until eggs are done to your liking and cheese is melted.

2 servings @ 3.5 grams of usable carbs each.

Salsa Scramble

Servings: 2

6 large Eggs
3 Tablespoons Water
1/4 teaspoon Salt
1 Tablespoon Butter
3 Tablespoons Salsa (any brand with no more than 3 grams of carbs per
    2 Tablespoons)
1/2 cup Cheddar or Monterrey Jack Cheese, shredded

Heat a 10" heavy, non-stick skillet over medium heat for 2 minutes. Add butter and swish to cover bottom of pan. Whisk eggs, water, and salt in a medium bowl until light and fluffy.

When butter is bubbling but not brown, pour in egg mixture and reduce heat to low. Cook and lift and fold until eggs are nearly set.

Add salsa and continue cooking and lifting until eggs are set but moist. Sprinkle with cheese, cover and turn off heat. Serve when cheese is melted.

2 servings @ 3.5 grams of usable carbs each.

Swiss Eggs & Sausage

Servings: 2

6 large Eggs
1 Tablespoon Butter
4 Tablespoons Red or Green Bell Pepper, chopped,
2 Tablespoons Onion, coarsely chopped
4 ounces fully cooked Smoked Sausage, sliced into 1/4" slices, remove casing, (no more than 1 gram of carbs per 2 ounces)
2 slices Swiss Cheese (Kraft® Swiss comes in the long package)
2 Tablespoons Water
Salt and Pepper to taste

Break eggs into medium bowl and set aside. Heat a heavy, 10" non-stick skillet over low heat for about 3 minutes. Add butter and melt, swishing to cover bottom of pan.

Sauté peppers, onions, and sausage until onions are translucent, about 3-4 minutes.

Lay cheese over mixture and cover until cheese melts. Remove cover and gently pour eggs over cheese, taking care not to break yolks. Cover and cook until eggs are done as desired, adding water when eggs are nearly done to steam the tops. Replace cover immediately to hold in steam. Salt and pepper to taste.

2 generous servings @ 3.4 grams of usable carbs each.

Taco Omelets

Servings: 2

6 large Eggs
1/4 cup Water
3/4 teaspoon Salt
1 Tablespoon Butter
1 cup Taco Meat (page 83)
1/2 cup Cheddar Cheese, shredded

Toppings (optional)
1 cup Lettuce
1/2 cup Tomato, chopped
1/4 cup Onion, chopped
4 Tablespoons Salsa (no more than 3 grams of carbs per 2 Tablespoons)
4 Tablespoons Sour Cream

Melt butter in an 8" heavy, non-stick skillet over medium-low heat for about 3 minutes, swishing to cover bottom of pan. Whisk eggs with water and salt until fluffy. Add 1/2 of the eggs and cover for 15-20 seconds.

Remove lid and lift eggs, letting uncooked portion flow underneath until set. Spoon 1/2 cup taco meat on one side, then 1/2 the cheese. Carefully fold in half and place on plate.

Keep warm while repeating with remaining eggs, taco meat, and cheese. Top with any or all desired toppings.

Note: Don't be afraid to add a little Jalapeño or Tabasco Sauce for some zip.

2 servings @ 1.8 grams of usable carbs each without toppings.

2 servings @ 8.5 grams of usable carbs each with toppings.

SOUPS

Chili 46

Cream Of Broccoli Soup 47

Ham & Asparagus Soup 48

Oyster Stew 49

Turkey Egg Drop Soup 50

Chili

Servings: 4

1 Tablespoon Cooking Oil
3/4 cup Onion, chopped
2 pounds Ground Beef, lean, coarse ground if possible
3/4 teaspoon Salt
1 Tablespoon bottled fresh minced Garlic, or equivalent fresh Garlic, minced
4 1/2 teaspoons Chili Powder
1 1/2 teaspoons Ground Cumin
1 cup canned Tomatoes with Juice
1 cup Water
2 cups Daikon Radish, peeled and cubed

In a 3 quart heavy saucepan, sauté onion in oil over low heat until translucent, about 3 minutes. Add ground beef and cook over high heat, stirring and breaking up with a spoon until browned and no pink remains.

Add remaining ingredients and simmer until Daikon radish is tender.

Serve with shredded cheddar cheese, chopped onions, and sour cream if desired.

Note: Toppings are figured on 1/4 cup of Cheddar Cheese, 2 Tablespoons of onion, and 2 Tablespoons of Sour Cream per serving.

4 servings @ 4.2 grams of usable carbs each without toppings.

4 servings @ 8.1 grams of usable carbs each with toppings.

Cream of Broccoli Soup

Servings: 4

1 Tablespoon Butter
2 Tablespoons Onion, chopped
1 – 14.5 ounce can Chicken Broth
1 pound Broccoli flowerets, trimmed and cut up
1 1/2 teaspoons Salt
1 teaspoon Garlic Salt
1 cup Heavy Whipping Cream
1/2 teaspoon Xanthan Gum

In a 3 quart heavy saucepan, sauté onions in butter over low heat until softened but not browned, about 3 minutes.

Add chicken broth and bring to a boil. Add broccoli, salt, and garlic salt and reduce heat to low and cook covered until soft, about 15 minutes.

Add heavy whipping cream and heat through. Do NOT boil. SLOWLY sprinkle Xanthan Gum and whisk in until thickened. Serve hot.

Note: Xanthan Gum acts as a thickener and can be found at most health food stores and some grocery stores.

4 servings @ 3.6 grams of usable carbs each.

Ham & Asparagus Soup

Servings: 5

1 – 14.5 ounce can Chicken Broth
1 pound fresh Asparagus, tough ends snapped off, washed and
   trimmed into 1/2" slices
1/4 teaspoon Salt
2 Tablespoons Butter
3 Tablespoons Onion, chopped
3 cups Ham, chopped (0 carbs)
3/4 cup Heavy Whipping Cream
1/2 cup Water
1/2 teaspoon Xanthan Gum
Salt and Pepper to taste

In a 3 quart saucepan bring chicken broth to a boil over high heat. Add asparagus and salt. Bring to a boil again, reduce heat, cover and simmer until asparagus is tender, about 10-15 minutes. Remove from heat. Remove and set aside 1/2 cup asparagus. Place rest of asparagus and broth in blender container and blend until smooth. Set aside. Wash and dry saucepan.

In same saucepan, melt butter over medium-low heat, add onion and sauté until soft, about 2-3 minutes. Add ham and sauté another 3 minutes, stirring frequently. Add reserved 1/2 cup asparagus.

Add blended broth mixture to ham, asparagus, and onions. Add cream and water and continue to heat but do not boil. Sprinkle with Xanthan Gum and stir briskly to thicken. Salt and pepper to taste. Heat another few minutes until thickened. Makes 5 – 1/2 cup servings.

Note: Do not add more Xanthan Gum. It will thicken in a few minutes. Xanthan Gum can be found in most health food stores and some grocery stores.

5 servings @ 3.8 grams of usable carbs each.

Oyster Stew

Servings: 3

2/3 cup Heavy Whipping Cream
3/4 cup Water
1   pint Oysters, fresh shucked with liquid
1   Tablespoon Butter
Salt and Pepper to taste

Heat heavy whipping cream and water over medium heat in a medium saucepan until very hot but not boiling.

When beginning to get quite warm, add oysters to cream mixture. Heat oysters until edges curl.

Do NOT overcook or the oysters will be tough.

Add butter and salt and pepper to taste.

Note: So delicious on a chilly day.

3 servings @ 8 grams of usable carbs each.

Turkey Egg Drop Soup
Servings: 6

3 cups Turkey Broth, leftover from Roast Turkey or Turkey Breast
1 – 14.5 ounce can Chicken Broth, ready to use (not concentrated)
1/2 cup Celery, chopped
Cooked Turkey, any amount, cut in chunks (make it as meaty as you like)
2 large Eggs, beaten
Kikkoman® Soy Sauce to taste
Salt and Pepper to taste
2 medium Green Onions, sliced with tops

Combine broths in a 3 1/2 quart sauce pan, cover and bring to a boil over medium heat. Add celery and turkey and reduce heat to low, cover and cook until celery is tender. Increase heat to high, bring to a boil and slowly pour in beaten eggs, stirring constantly until eggs are set in shreds.

Season with Kikkoman® soy sauce. Salt and pepper to taste. Start with soy sauce since it is very salty. Add green onions just before serving.

Note: You can try this recipe with leftover chicken. You'll be surprised how great it tastes.

6 servings @ .8 grams of usable carbs each.

SALADS & SALAD DRESSINGS

Cabbage & Bacon Salad 52

Confetti Salad 53

Creamy Cole Slaw 54

Dilled Creamed Cucumbers 55

Grilled Chicken Salad With Vegetables 56

Pork Salad 57

Roast Beef Salad 58

Sweet Cauliflower And Bacon Salad 59

Taco Salad 60

Turkey Salad 61

Mediterranean Chicken Salad 62

Bleu Cheese Dressing 63

Ranch Dressing 64

Red French Dressing 65

Sun-Dried Tomato-Mushroom Vinaigrette Dressing 66

Sweet Mayonnaise For Miracle Whip Lovers 67

Thousand Island Dressing 68

Cabbage & Bacon Salad

Servings: 6

1 - 1 pound head of Cabbage, chopped small or shredded
1/2 medium Red or Green Bell Pepper, chopped
3 Tablespoons Celery, chopped
1/2 cup Cooking Oil
1/3 cup Rice Vinegar (do not substitute)
4 Tablespoons Splenda®, sugar substitute
1/4 teaspoon dry Mustard
1/2 teaspoon McCormick® Onion Juice (found in spice section of supermarket)
1/2 teaspoon Black Pepper
3 Tablespoons bottled or packaged Real Bacon Bits (0 carbs)

Mix cabbage, peppers, and celery in medium bowl with tight fitting lid. Mix remaining ingredients in a small bowl and pour over vegetables.

Mix well and refrigerate several hours to blend flavors.

6 servings @ 3.3 grams of usable carbs each.

Confetti Salad

Servings: 5

1 - 14.5 ounce can French Style Green Beans, drained
1 cup fresh Tomatoes, seeded and chopped
1/4 cup Onion, chopped fine
6 large Ripe Olives, cut in thin strips
1 1/2 inch block of Real American Cheese (not Velveeta®), about 2
     ounces, cut into1/4" cubes
1/4 cup Mayonnaise (0 carbs)
1/2 teaspoon Splenda®, sugar substitute
1/8 teaspoon Salt
1/8 teaspoon Pepper
5 cups Iceberg Lettuce, shredded

Toss all ingredients, except lettuce, gently together. Refrigerate until cold.
Arrange each serving over 1 cup shredded lettuce. Refrigerate leftovers.

Note: Try using Romaine instead of Iceberg Lettuce.

5 - 1/2 cup servings @ 4.6 grams of usable carbs each.

Creamy Cole Slaw

Servings: 10

4 cups Cabbage, chopped fine or shredded
2 Tablespoons Red or Green Bell Peppers, chopped fine
1/4 cup Heavy Whipping Cream
3/4 cup Mayonnaise (0 carbs)
4 Tablespoons Splenda®, sugar substitute
1/4 teaspoon Salt
Pepper to taste

Mix cabbage and bell pepper together in a large bowl. Whisk remaining ingredients together in a small bowl until smooth. Pour over cabbage and mix well.

Chill in refrigerator.

Note: This is a huge hit at every family gathering and every party we attend. I have more requests for this recipe than almost any other and it's so quick and easy!

10 - 1/2 cup servings @ 1.7 grams of usable carbs each.

Dilled Creamed Cucumbers

Servings: 8

1/2 cup Mayonnaise
1 1/4 cups Sour Cream
1 Tablespoon Splenda®, sugar substitute
2 Tablespoons Rice Vinegar (do not substitute)
1 teaspoon Dill Weed
2 teaspoons bottled fresh minced Garlic, or equivalent fresh Garlic, minced
1 teaspoon Salt
5 medium Cucumbers, peeled, sliced thin, salted well, and drained in colander for 30 minutes

Whisk all ingredients, except cucumbers, in a medium bowl. Rinse cucumbers well and pat dry with paper towels. Stir into dressing mixture.

Refrigerate and serve cold.

Note: When my friend, who hates cucumbers, told me this recipe was wonderful, I knew it would be a hit. Also, the usable carb count is considering that all of the dressing is consumed, which is usually not the case.

8 servings @ 4.6 grams of usable carbs each.

Grilled Chicken Salad with Vegetables

Servings: 2

2 or 4 Chicken Breast halves, boneless (depends on how hungry you are)
4 Tablespoons Olive Oil, divided
Garlic Salt to taste
1/2 medium Red Bell Pepper, cut in 1" strips
1/2 medium Green Bell Pepper, cut in 1" strips
1/4 medium Onion, cut in thick strips
1 medium Zucchini, sliced 1/4" thick
3 cups Lettuce, any variety
1/2 medium Tomato, cut into wedges
1/2 cup Cucumber, sliced 1/4" thick

Dressing:
1/3 cup Olive Oil
3 Tablespoons Rice Vinegar
1 teaspoon Splenda®, sugar substitute
1/2 teaspoon bottled fresh minced Garlic, or equivalent fresh Garlic, minced

Wash chicken breasts and pat dry with paper towels. Brush both sides with 2 Tablespoons of olive oil and sprinkle with garlic salt. Grill over medium coals or on gas grill. Turn every 2-3 minutes until juice runs clear. Keep warm. Note: The secret to juicy chicken is turning every 2-3 minutes.

Sauté peppers, onions, and zucchini in 2 Tablespoons of olive oil in a medium size heavy skillet until tender-crisp. Sprinkle lightly with garlic salt while sautéing. Remove from heat.

Arrange greens, cucumbers, and tomatoes on 2 large serving plates. Arrange sautéed vegetables on top. Slice chicken and place attractively on salads.

Dressing: Mix olive oil, rice vinegar, Splenda, and garlic. Drizzle over salads.

2 servings @ 9.6 grams of usable carbs each.

Pork Salad

Servings: 10

1   pound Pork Roast, cooked or leftover
3   Tablespoons Onion, chopped
1/4   cup Celery, diced
3/4   cup Mayonnaise or Sweet Mayonnaise recipe, (page 67)

Place all ingredients in food processor and process until desired consistency or chop roast, onion, and celery fine by hand, then stir in mayonnaise.

Note: This is so delicious by itself but also great on a leaf of Romaine lettuce or low carb roll or bread. Just be sure to count the extra carbs.

10 - 1/4 cup servings @ .2 grams of usable carbs each.

Roast Beef Salad

Servings: 7

1 pound leftover Roast Beef, trim fat and cut in 1" pieces
1/2 cup Onion, coarsely chopped
1/2 cup Celery, coarsely chopped
1 medium Dill Pickle, coarsely chopped
1 cup Mayonnaise or Sweet Mayonnaise recipe, (page 67)

Place roast beef in food processor bowl and chop into small pieces. Add remaining ingredients except for mayonnaise.

Process until desired consistency. Add mayonnaise and mix well.

If you don't have a food processor, you can grind meat in a grinder and chop remaining ingredients.

Note: Also wonderful on a leaf of Romaine lettuce or low carb roll or bread. Just be sure to count the extra carbs.

7 - 1/2 cup servings @ 1.1 grams of usable carbs each.

Sweet Cauliflower & Bacon Salad

Servings: 10

1 medium head of Cauliflower, cut into 1" flowerets
2 cups Water
1 Tablespoon Salt

Dressing:
1/2 cup Mayonnaise
1/4 cup Heavy Whipping Cream
2 Tablespoons Splenda®, sugar substitute
3 Tablespoons Red or Green Bell Pepper, chopped
2 Tablespoons Onion, chopped fine
3/4 teaspoon Salt
Pepper to taste
5 strips Bacon, fried crisp, drained and crumbled or equivalent jarred
   Real Bacon pieces

Bring water to a boil in large saucepan. Add cauliflower, then sprinkle with salt. Cover and bring to full boil again. Boil 1 minute, drain in colander, then return to pan and rinse in cold water until cool.

Drain and place in large mixing bowl. Set aside.

Whisk mayonnaise and heavy whipping cream in a small bowl until smooth. Add remaining dressing ingredients and whisk. Pour over cauliflower and toss. Refrigerate several hours before serving.

Note: Real Bacon pieces are located in salad dressing aisle near the croutons.

10 - 1/2 cup servings @ 1.6 grams of usable carbs each.

Taco Salad

Servings: 2

4 cups Romaine Lettuce, coarsely chopped
2 cups Taco Meat recipe, (page 83)
1 cup Cheddar Cheese, shredded
2 Tablespoons Onion, sliced thin lengthwise
8 Cherry Tomatoes, halved
4 large Ripe Olives, sliced
1/3 cup Mayonnaise (0 carbs)
3 Tablespoons Salsa (no more than 3 grams of carbs per 2 Tablespoons)
Pinch of Salt
2 or 3 sprigs of Cilantro Leaves, whole
Sour Cream (optional)

Arrange greens on 2 large plates. Top with taco meat, then next 4 ingredients in order given. Arrange attractively.

Mix mayo, salsa, salt, and cilantro leaves. Spoon over salads evenly.

Note: If you like it hot just add some Tabasco or seeded Jalapeños and if topping with sour cream be sure to count the extra carbs.

2 servings @ 8.1 grams of usable carbs each.

Turkey Salad
Servings: 6

4 cups cooked, leftover Turkey, chopped
1 stalk Celery, about 9", chopped
2 medium Green Onions, sliced, including tops
3 Tablespoons slivered Almonds, toasted (optional)
3/4 cup Mayonnaise or Sweet Mayonnaise recipe, (page 67)
1/4 cup Heavy Whipping Cream
Salt and Pepper, to taste

Mix all ingredients, except mayonnaise and heavy whipping cream, in a medium bowl. Whisk mayonnaise and heavy whipping cream together in a small bowl until smooth.

Pour over turkey mixture and mix until well combined. Refrigerate covered. Makes about 3 cups total.

Variation:
Chicken Salad
Substitute equal amounts of cooked Chicken for the Turkey. Proceed as directed.

Note: For the best flavor, combine white and dark meat. You'll be amazed at how much better the flavor is.

6 - 1/2 cup servings @ .9 grams of usable carbs each with slivered almonds.

6 - 1/2 cup servings @ .7 grams of usable carbs each without slivered almonds.

Mediterranean Chicken Salad

Servings: 2

2 fresh boneless, skinless Chicken Breasts
2 Tablespoons Olive Oil
Salt and Pepper, to taste
4 cups Romaine Leaves, coarsely shredded
1/2 cup Cherry Tomato halves
2 ounces Cream Cheese, cut in 1/2" cubes
1/4 cup Ripe Olives, sliced
1/4 cup Green Onions, sliced in 1/2" lengths
1/2 cup Sun-Dried Tomato Mushroom Vinaigrette recipe, (page 66)
Freshly shredded Parmesan Cheese for garnish (optional)

Wash chicken and pat dry with paper towels. Brush chicken breasts with olive oil on all sides. Salt and pepper to taste.

Grill or broil until juices run clear when pierced with a knife. Set aside to cool a bit.

On 2 dinner plates, attractively divide remaining ingredients in order given, except Sun-Dried Tomato Mushroom Vinaigrette. Cut slightly cooled chicken in slices or chunks and arrange on salad.

Drizzle with Sun-Dried Tomato Mushroom Vinaigrette.

Note: This recipe is one of our favorites. Once you make this one you'll definitely want to share it with your guests. Be sure to count carbs in Parmesan Cheese if using.

2 servings @ 9.3 grams of usable carbs each.

Bleu Cheese Dressing

2/3 cup Mayonnaise
2/3 cup Heavy Whipping Cream
1/4 cup Buttermilk
1 1/2 teaspoons bottled fresh minced Garlic, or equivalent fresh Garlic,
    minced
1/2 teaspoon Garlic Powder
1/8 teaspoon Salt
1/2 teaspoon Splenda®, sugar substitute
1 - 4 ounce package crumbled Bleu Cheese

Whisk all ingredients, except bleu cheese, together in a medium bowl.

Stir in bleu cheese. Pour about 1/2 of mixture into a blender and purée. Stir purée back into remaining mixture and refrigerate.

Makes about 2 cups total.

1 Tablespoon @ .4 grams of usable carbs each.

Ranch Dressing

Servings: 32

1 cup Mayonnaise (0 carbs)
1 cup Buttermilk
3/4 teaspoon Cavenders® Greek Seasoning or any brand of Greek
     Seasoning
1/4 teaspoon Garlic Salt with Parsley
1/4 teaspoon Splenda®, sugar substitute
Few grinds of Pepper
Pinch Xanthan Gum

Whisk all ingredients until smooth and then refrigerate.

Note: Please remember that it only takes a small amount of Xanthan Gum to
thicken a recipe. Will get thicker as it stands. Always shake well before
serving.

Makes 2 cups @ .4 grams of usable carbs per Tablespoon.

Red French Dressing

Servings: 32

1 cup Hunts® Tomato Sauce
1/4 cup White Vinegar
1/2 cup plus 2 Tablespoons Splenda®, sugar substitute
2 Tablespoons Onion, chopped
1 clove fresh Garlic, minced or equivalent bottled fresh minced Garlic
1 teaspoon dry Mustard
1 cup Cooking Oil
Pinch Xanthan Gum

Place all ingredients, except Xanthan Gum and cooking oil, in blender container. Blend until onion and garlic are liquefied.

While blender is running on medium speed, add cooking oil very slowly, in 1/8" stream, will take a few minutes. When oil is incorporated, continue blending another 30 seconds.

Add pinch Xanthan Gum, blend a few seconds. Makes 3 cups of dressing. Refrigerate covered.

Note: *Always shake well before serving.*

1 Tablespoon @ .5 grams of usable carbs each.

Sun-Dried Tomato Mushroom Vinaigrette

Servings: 18

6 Sun-Dried Tomatoes, not in oil, snipped with scissors into small pieces
1/3 cup boiling Water
1 - 7 ounce can Mushroom Stems and Pieces, drained and chopped
3 cloves fresh Garlic, minced or equivalent bottled fresh minced Garlic
   (do not use Garlic Powder or Garlic Salt)
1/2 cup Extra Virgin Olive Oil
1 cup Canola Oil
1/4 teaspoon Salt
1/4 cup Balsamic Vinegar
1/4 cup White Vinegar
1 Tablespoon Splenda®, sugar substitute
1/2 teaspoon dried Oregano Powder

Pour boiling water over sun-dried tomatoes in a small bowl. Let set for 20 minutes, then drain well.

Mix all ingredients together and place in a covered container.

Note: Stir well before serving each time. Keeps well in the refrigerator.

18 - 2 Tablespoon servings @ 1 gram of usable carbs each.

Sweet Mayonnaise for Miracle Whip Lovers!

1 quart Mayonnaise (0 carbs)
1/4 cup Splenda®, sugar substitute

Spoon mayonnaise into medium mixing bowl. Whisk in Splenda® until well combined.

Spoon back into jar and label "Sweet".

Note: So quick and easy to make and it's lower in carbs than regular Miracle Whip®.

1 Tablespoon serving @ a trace of usable carbs each.

Thousand Island Dressing

1 cup Mayonnaise (0 carbs)
2 Tablespoons Heavy Whipping Cream
1/4 cup Nancy's Ketchup recipe, (page 125) or any equivalent low carb
    Ketchup
1 Tablespoon Dill Pickle, chopped fine and well drained
1 Tablespoon Onion, minced
2 small Pimiento-Stuffed Green Olives, chopped
1 hard-cooked Egg, chopped fine

Combine all ingredients and stir until well mixed. Store in refrigerator.

Makes about 1 3/4 cups.

Note: Not only is this dressing great on your favorite salads, but wait until you
    try it on the Reuben Balls Variation recipe, (page 16).

1 Tablespoon @ .2 grams of usable carbs each.

ENTREES

BEEF

Chicken Fried Steak... 70
Ground Beef And Cabbage Casserole........................... 71
Hamburger Mushroom And Green Bean Casserole 72
Baked Italian Deli Sandwich 73
Meatballs Alfredo... 74
Mexi Stuffed Peppers 75
Mexican Pizza 76
Mexican Pizza Crust 77
Old-Fashioned Meatloaf....................................... 78
Pizza Roll Meatloaf 79
Prime Rib With Mushroom Au Jus.............................. 80
Quick Chow Mein 81
Rueben Lasagna 82
Taco Meat... 83

PORK

Quick Hot Deli Plate... 84
BBQ Ribs 85
Fresh Pork With Sauerkraut Cabbage And Tomatoes 86
Fried Smoked Sausage 87
Ham Patties 88
Pizza... 89
Pizza Crust... 90
Pork And Cabbage With Sauerkraut 91
Pork Chops With Cream Gravy 92
Sweet And Sour Pork... 99
Sweet And Sour Pork Vegetable Stir-Fry 93
Zucchini Boats 94

POULTRY

Chicken Cacciatore... 95
Chicken Olé 96
Chicken Parmigiana.. 97
Quick Swiss Chicken With Broccoli........................... 98
Sweet And Sour Chicken...................................... 99

FISH & SEAFOOD

Broiled Halibut With Citrus Dill Butter 100
Crispy Fried Fish.. 101
Crusty Cajun Salmon With Cajun Mayonnaise 102
Greek Baked Salmon 103
Salmon Patties.. 104
Shrimp Scampi Parmesano 105
Sweet And Sour Shrimp 99

Chicken Fried Steak

Servings: 3

3/4 cup Pork Rinds, plain or spicy, crushed fine
3 Tablespoons Atkins® Bake Mix
1 1/2 teaspoons Seasoned Salt
1 large Egg, beaten
2 pounds Beef Cube Steaks
4 Tablespoons Cooking Oil
Salt and Pepper to taste

Cream Gravy:
1 1/2 cups Heavy Whipping Cream
1/2 teaspoon Xanthan Gum
Salt and Pepper to taste

Breading:
Mix pork rinds, bake mix, and seasoned salt in a large, shallow dish. A pie pan works well. Set aside.

Beat egg in another large, shallow dish.

Dip cube steaks in egg, then breading, shaking off excess. Lay in single layer on waxed paper or foil.

Pre-heat oven to 225°

Heat oil in a large, heavy non-stick skillet until hot but not smoking. Fry in 2 batches if necessary, adding more oil if needed, until browned on both sides. Keep warm uncovered in 225° oven.

Gravy:
Pour off excess oil and add heavy whipping cream to skillet. Bring to a boil, scraping any browned bits from the bottom of the pan. Sprinkle Xanthan Gum over and stir well until thickened.

Add salt and pepper to taste. Pour over steaks and serve immediately.

3 servings @ 4.6 grams of usable carbs each.

EAT YOURSELF THIN LIKE I DID!

Ground Beef & Cabbage Casserole

Servings: 8

1 Tablespoon Cooking Oil
1/4 cup Onion, chopped
2 pounds lean Ground Beef
2 teaspoons Salt, divided
1 teaspoon Garlic Powder
1 - 1 1/2 pound head of Cabbage, cored and cut into 1" pieces
2 Tablespoons Tomato Paste
3/4 cup Water

Sauté onion in cooking oil over medium-low heat in a large, deep heavy skillet about 2 minutes. Crumble ground beef into pan, increase heat to medium-high, add 1 teaspoon salt and garlic powder. Cook and stir, breaking meat into small pieces with the back of a spoon, until no pink remains.

Decrease heat to medium-low, add cabbage, remaining salt, and tomato paste and mix well. Add water and mix well. Simmer covered over low heat until cabbage is as done as you like.

Serve hot. Also reheats very well.

8 - 1 cup servings @ 3.6 grams of usable carbs each.

Hamburger Mushroom & Green Bean Casserole

Servings: 5

1 teaspoon Cooking Oil
1/2 cup Onion, chopped
1/2 cup Celery, chopped
2 pounds lean Ground Beef
2 teaspoons Garlic Salt
1 teaspoon Salt
1/2 teaspoon Pepper
2 1/4 cups fresh or frozen Cut Green Beans
3/4 cup Heavy Whipping Cream
1 - 7 ounce can Mushroom Stems and Pieces, undrained
1 1/2 teaspoons instant Beef Bouillon Granules
1/2 teaspoon Xanthan Gum
2 teaspoons Kikkoman® Soy Sauce
1/4 cup sliced Water Chestnuts, cut in strips

In a large, deep heavy skillet, sauté onion and celery in cooking oil over medium-low heat, about 3-4 minutes until onion is tender. Add crumbled ground beef, garlic salt, salt, and pepper. Increase heat to high and brown, breaking up with the back of a spoon and stirring often until no pink remains. Drain fat. Add green beans and reduce heat to low. Cover and simmer while preparing sauce.

Measure heavy whipping cream into a bowl or large measuring cup. Drain mushroom liquid into heavy whipping cream. Add bouillon granules and mix well. Whisk in Xanthan gum then mushrooms.

Stir into ground beef mixture and add soy sauce. Cover and simmer about 20 minutes or until green beans are as done as you prefer. Stir in water chestnuts and heat through.

Note: Xanthan Gum can be found in nearly every health food store and it works great as a thickening agent. Always remember that a little goes a long way.

5 servings @ 6 grams of usable carbs each.

Baked Italian Deli Sandwich

Servings: 4

4 large Eggs, separated
1/4 teaspoon Cream of Tartar
1 Tablespoon Atkins® Bake Mix
1 Tablespoon liquid from Marinated Artichoke Hearts
1/4 teaspoon Salt
2 teaspoons bottled fresh minced Garlic or equivalent fresh Garlic, minced
1 teaspoon dried Basil Leaves
1/4 teaspoon Xanthan Gum
1/4 teaspoon Guar Gum
1 pound deli Italian Roast Beef, shaved (if unavailable use regular Roast Beef or Cajun Roast Beef)
1 - 6 ounce jar Marinated Artichoke Hearts, drained
(reserve 1 Tablespoon liquid for batter, as mentioned above)
6 ounces Hot Pepper Cheese, sliced
1/4 medium Onion, sliced thin

Pre-heat oven to 350°

Butter an 8" round or square cake non-stick pan. Place egg whites and cream of tartar in a medium bowl. Set aside.

In another medium bowl whisk egg yolks and next 7 ingredients together. Set aside. Whip egg whites and cream of tartar with an electric mixer until stiff but not dry. Gently fold in egg yolk mixture. Pour 1/2 of batter into buttered pan.

Bake 10 minutes @ 350°. Remove from oven and layer remaining ingredients in order given. Top with remaining batter. Bake about 25 minutes or until browned and springs back when touched with a finger.

4 servings @ 6.3 grams of usable carbs each.

Meatballs Alfredo

Servings: 18

1 pound extra lean Ground Beef
1 pound Italian Sausage (I use Jimmy Dean® brand)
1/4 cup Onion, chopped fine
2 teaspoons bottled fresh minced Garlic or equivalent fresh Garlic,
    minced
1/2 teaspoon Salt
1 large Egg
1/2 cup Water
1/2 teaspoon dried Basil Leaves
1/2 teaspoon dried Oregano Leaves
1 teaspoon Fennel Seed
Pinch crushed Red Pepper (optional)
1 - recipe Nancy's Alfredo Sauce, (page 121)

Pre-heat oven to 350°

Mix all ingredients together, except Alfredo Sauce, in a large mixing bowl with hands until well combined. Pat into a square on a piece of waxed paper or plastic wrap.

Cut into 18 equal pieces and form each into a ball and place on a large sprayed baking pan with sides. Bake @ 350° for 45-50 minutes.

Make Alfredo Sauce about 10 minutes before meatballs are done. Place meatballs in serving dish and pour Alfredo Sauce over meatballs and garnish with parsley if desired.

Note: Sprinkle with a little crushed Red Pepper for some zip.

18 servings @ 1.2 grams of usable carbs each.

Mexi Stuffed Peppers
Servings: 6

3 medium Red or Green Bell Peppers
2 pounds lean Ground Beef
2 large Eggs
3/4 cup Water
1 Tablespoon bottled fresh minced Garlic or equivalent fresh Garlic, minced
1/4 cup Onion, chopped fine
1 Tablespoon Chili Powder
2 Tablespoons Salsa (any brand no more than 3 grams of carbs per 2 Tablespoons)
2 teaspoons Salt
1 1/2 cups Cheddar Cheese, shredded

Pre-heat oven to 350°

Wash peppers, cut in half and remove seeds and veins. Mix remaining ingredients, except cheddar cheese, with your hands until well combined. Divide into 6 equal portions and stuff pepper halves with mixture.

Place in baking pan with sides, large enough to hold in 1 layer. Pour 1/4 cup water in bottom of pan. Cover with foil and bake @ 350° for 45-55 minutes or until cooked through.

Remove foil and sprinkle each with 1/4 cup cheddar cheese. Return to oven uncovered 10 minutes. Serve hot.

6 servings @ 5 grams of usable carbs each.

Mexican Pizza
Servings: 8

1 - recipe Mexican Pizza Crust (page 77)

Mexican Pizza Sauce:
2 Tablespoons Tomato Paste
2 Tablespoons Salsa
1/4 cup Water
1 teaspoon Garlic Powder
1/2 teaspoon Ground Cumin

Topping:
1 pound Extra Lean Ground Beef
3/4 teaspoon Salt
1 1/2 teaspoons Chili Powder
1/2 teaspoon Garlic Powder
1/2 cup Ripe Olives, sliced
6 whole Jalapeños, seeded, sliced, and chopped (optional)
4 Tablespoons Onion, chopped
12 ounce package Cheddar Cheese, shredded

Mexican Pizza Sauce
Mix all ingredients together in a medium bowl and spread evenly on crust. Set aside.

Topping
Brown ground beef and seasonings in a medium non-stick skillet until no pink remains, breaking up with a spoon into small chunks. Drain well and spread evenly over crust. Top with olives, jalapeños, onions, and then cheese.

Bake @ 425° for 10-12 minutes or until cheese is melted.

8 servings @ 4.7 grams of usable carbs each with Jalapeños.

8 servings @ 4.3 grams of usable carbs each without Jalapeños.

Mexican Pizza Crust

Servings: 8

3/4 cup Warm Water
1 can Keto® Pizza Dough Mix
1 teaspoon Olive Oil
1 packet Yeast (included in dough mix)
1/4 teaspoon Garlic Powder
1 teaspoon Chili Powder
1/2 teaspoon Ground Cumin

Place all ingredients in bread machine in order given. Start machine on dough cycle. If too dry after a minute or so, add water a teaspoon at a time. If your bread machine does not have a dough cycle use regular setting and remove dough after first kneading. If you do not have a bread machine, combine ingredients in a medium bowl and knead until smooth, about 10 minutes. Roll out to about a 14" circle or rectangle if you prefer. I roll it as thin as possible.

Pre-heat oven to 400°

Place on well oiled pizza pan or jelly roll pan. Bake for 10 minutes. Remove from oven and cool for 5 minutes before adding toppings.

Increase oven to 425°.

8 servings @ 2 grams of usable carbs each.

Old-Fashioned Meatloaf

Servings: 8

2 pounds lean Ground Beef
3/4 cup Water
1 teaspoon Salt
1/2 teaspoon Pepper
1 large Egg
1 teaspoon bottled fresh minced Garlic or equivalent fresh Garlic, minced
3/4 cup Nancy's Ketchup recipe, (page 125) or equivalent low carb Ketchup, divided
1/2 cup Onion, chopped fine

Pre-heat oven to 350°

Mix all ingredients including 4 Tablespoons of ketchup together with hands until well combined. Shape into a loaf and place in a sprayed 9"x13" pan. Spread remaining ketchup on top.

Bake @ 350° for 75-90 minutes or until done.

Note: My family and friends go crazy over this favorite, I think yours will too.

8 servings @ 1.8 grams of usable carbs each.

Pizza Roll Meatloaf

Servings: 8

2 pounds extra lean Ground Beef
1/4 cup Onion, chopped
3 teaspoons bottled fresh minced Garlic or equivalent fresh Garlic,
    minced and divided
1 1/2 teaspoons dried Basil Leaves, divided
1 1/2 teaspoons Oregano Leaves, divided
1 teaspoon Fennel Seed
1/2 teaspoon crushed Red Pepper, divided (optional)
2 1/8 teaspoons Salt
1/2 cup plus 2 Tablespoons Water, divided
2 Tablespoons Tomato Paste
1/4 cup Parmesan Cheese, grated
8 ounce package Mozzarella Cheese, sliced
1/2 cup fresh Mushrooms, chopped or a 4 ounce can of Mushroom
    slices, drained
1/2 cup Pepperoni slices

Pre-heat oven to 350°

Mix ground beef, onion, 2 teaspoons garlic, 1 teaspoon basil, 1 teaspoon oregano, fennel seed, salt, crushed red pepper if using, and 1/2 cup water. Mix well with hands until well blended.

Shape into a 10"x14" rectangle on waxed paper or plastic wrap.

Set aside.

Mix tomato paste, remaining garlic, basil, oregano, and remaining 2 Tablespoons water. Spread evenly over meat. Sprinkle parmesan evenly over sauce, lay mozzarella slices over parmesan cheese. Top with pepperoni slices, then mushrooms.

Carefully roll meat from 10" side into a roll resembling a cake roll, using waxed paper or plastic wrap to help roll along. Seal seam by pinching together well and seal ends by pinching together so cheese will not leak out.

Bake 1 hour @ 350°. Let stand loosely covered with aluminum foil for 10 minutes before slicing into 8 equal slices.

8 servings @ 2.3 grams of usable carbs each.

Prime Rib with Mushroom Au Jus

Servings: 6

3 1/2 pound Beef Rib Roast, chine bone removed
1 Tablespoon Schilling® Montreal Steak Seasoning, original or spicy
2 teaspoons bottled fresh minced Garlic or 4 cloves fresh Garlic, minced
1 double recipe Marvelous Mushrooms recipe, (page 114)

Au Jus:
2 cups Beef Broth or Beef Bouillon
1 teaspoon bottled fresh minced Garlic or 2 cloves fresh Garlic, minced
1 Tablespoon plus 1 teaspoon Kikkoman® Soy Sauce
2 teaspoons Worcestershire Sauce (0 carbs)

Pre-heat oven to 325°

Trim excess fat from outer edge of roast. Rub all sides with garlic, then sprinkle all sides with Montreal Steak Seasoning, pressing it into the meat. Place bone side down into sprayed roaster with at least 2 sides.

Roast until desired doneness. I use a meat thermometer and remove it from the oven when it is 5 degrees below desired temperature. If you do not have a meat thermometer, roast approximately 2 hours for Rare, 2 1/2 hours for Medium, and 3 1/2 hours for Well done. While meat is roasting prepare Marvelous Mushrooms recipe, (page 114).

When meat is desired doneness, remove and place on cutting board and let stand for 15 minutes covered loosely with aluminum foil before carving. While meat is standing, make Au Jus and add mushrooms. Heat until very hot.

Au Jus:
Mix all ingredients in a medium bowl and add to drippings in roaster. Bring to a boil, scraping browned bits from pan. Slice roast and ladle Au Jus over or around each serving.

Note: You may omit mushrooms if you don't care for them.

6 servings @ 1.6 grams of usable carbs each with mushrooms.

6 servings @ 1 gram of usable carbs each without mushrooms.

Quick Chow Mein

Servings: 4

2 pounds Ground Beef or Chow Mein meat (available at some markets)
Salt to taste
1 teaspoon bottled fresh minced Garlic or equivalent fresh Garlic, minced
3 cups Celery, sliced 1/3" thick
1/2 medium Onion, sliced lengthwise (about 3 ounces)
1 cup Beef Broth or Beef Bouillon
1 - 7 ounce can Mushrooms, sliced or Stems and Pieces, drained
1 - 8 ounce can Bamboo Shoots, drained, rinsed with water and drained
1 - 6 ounce can Dawn Fresh® Mushroom Steak Sauce (in a small, yellow can usually found near bottled Steak Sauce)
3 Tablespoons Kikkoman® Soy Sauce
1/2 teaspoon Xanthan Gum
Salt and Pepper to taste

Brown ground beef or chow mein meat and salt in a non-stick, heavy 4 quart saucepan over medium-high heat, breaking up meat with a spoon and stirring frequently.

When browned and no pink remains, drain fat and discard. Add celery, onions, and beef broth and reduce heat to low. Cover and simmer until celery is tender.

Add remaining ingredients except Xanthan gum and continue to simmer until heated through. Sprinkle Xanthan gum over and stir until thickened.

Correct seasonings and serve.

Note: Reheats well. Great to make ahead for quick meals.

4 servings @ 6.1 grams of usable carbs each.

Rueben Lasagna

Servings: 4

1 cup Sauerkraut, liquid squeezed out
1/2 cup Sour Cream
1 pound Corned Beef deli meat, sliced very thin
8 ounces Swiss Cheese, sliced
2 Tablespoons Onion, finely chopped
1/4 teaspoon Caraway Seed (optional)

Pre-heat oven to 350°

Mix sauerkraut and sour cream together. Spray an 8" square baking pan. Layer 1/2 of corned beef on bottom. Cover with layer of swiss cheese, then carefully spread 1/2 of sauerkraut mixture over swiss cheese. Sprinkle with all of the onions.

Repeat layers ending with sauerkraut. Sprinkle with caraway seed if desired.

Bake @ 350° for 35-40 minutes. Serve hot.

Note: I like to use Vlasic® or Claussen® brand of sauerkraut. Claussen® is found in the refrigerated section.

4 large servings @ 5.3 grams of usable carbs each.

Taco Meat

2 pounds lean ground Beef
2 teaspoons Garlic Salt
2 Tablespoons Chili Powder
1 teaspoon ground Cumin
1 teaspoon Salt

Brown ground beef over medium-high heat in a large deep skillet with remaining ingredients, breaking meat up with a spoon. When no pink remains, remove from heat and drain any excess fat. Cool slightly.

Makes approximately 7 cups.

Use in Taco Salad recipe (page 60), Taco Omelet recipe (page 44), or Quick & Easy Tex-Mex Eggs recipe (page 41).

Note: You can use your own imagination to create some wonderful entrees with this quick and easy recipe. I like to make this one ahead of time and freeze it, that way I always have it available for a quick meal.

Whole recipe has a total of 4 grams of usable carbs.

Quick Hot Deli Plate

Servings: 2

1 pound deli meat - shaved Ham, Roast Beef, Corned Beef, Pastrami, Turkey, or a combination of your favorite deli meats. (Just make sure they are 0 carbs)

2 Tablespoons Green Olives, sliced

2 Tablespoons Ripe Olives, sliced

6 ounces Cheddar Cheese, Swiss, Hot Pepper, Mozzarella, or your favorite cheese, sliced

Divide all ingredients between 2 shallow soup plates sprayed with non-stick cooking spray. Layer in order given.

Cover each with a sprayed upside down paper plate. Microwave on medium until cheese melts.

Serve immediately.

Note: This has become a family favorite around our house. It's not only quick and easy, it's delicious too!

2 servings @ 6 grams of usable carbs each.

BBQ Ribs

Servings: 3

5 pounds Pork Spareribs, silverskin removed or at least cut through
Brisket Rub (I use Adams® brand)
1/2 cup Nancy's BBQ Sauce, recipe (page 122) or equivalent low carb
    BBQ Sauce

Rinse ribs and leave damp. Apply brisket rub and rub into meat. It takes about 2-3 Tablespoons or so.

Refrigerate in lock-top bag at least 8 hours. Preferably overnight but no longer.

Pre-heat oven to 275°

Place ribs in single layer in a large, sprayed baking pan or two with sides. Bake @ 275° for 3 hours or until very tender. Baste with BBQ sauce the last hour.

Note: *Silverskin is located on the underside.*

3 generous servings @ 4 grams of usable carbs each.

Fresh Pork with Sauerkraut Cabbage and Tomatoes

Servings: 6

2 1/2 pounds boneless Pork Top Loin Chops or Roast,
   cut into 1/2" thick pieces
1 teaspoon Cooking Oil
6 slices Bacon, cut in 1/2" pieces
1/2 cup Onion, chopped
2 cups Sauerkraut
2 1/2 cups Cabbage, shredded
1 cup canned Tomatoes, broken up with juice
1/8 teaspoon Pepper
1 teaspoon Brown Sugar Twin®, sugar substitute
1/4 cup Water
Salt to taste

Pre-heat oven to 325°

Heat large, deep oven-proof skillet over medium-high heat, brushed with oil. When hot, brown pork in a single layer on both sides. Transfer to a plate and set aside.

Lower heat and fry bacon for 2 minutes. Add onions and continue frying until onions are softened, about 2-3 minutes. Add remaining ingredients, except pork, mix well and simmer over low heat until cabbage is limp. Add pork and bury it as much as possible in mixture.

Bake covered @ 325° for 45 minutes to an hour.

Note: Watch for a big difference in carb counts on different brands of sauerkraut. I use Vlasic® or Claussen®. Claussen® is found in the refrigerated section. This is even better the next day when reheated. Also, this dish is wonderful with a dab of sour cream, just be sure to count the extra carbs.

6 servings @ 2.8 grams of usable carbs each.

Fried Smoked Sausage

Servings: 3

2 pounds Smoked Sausage (fully cooked and no more than 1 gram of
   carbs per 2 ounces)
1 large Egg, beaten
1 cup Pork Rinds, crushed fine (plain or spicy)
2 Tablespoons Atkins® Bake Mix
1/2 teaspoon Garlic Powder
1/4 cup Cooking Oil

Remove casing from sausage and cut in 3" pieces. Cut each piece in half, lengthwise. Place egg in small bowl. Set aside.

Mix pork rinds, bake mix, and garlic powder in shallow dish. Set aside. Heat oil in a large heavy skillet over medium heat.

When hot, dip sausage pieces in egg, then pork rinds and fry turning until browned on all sides. Serve hot.

Note: Nancy's Ketchup recipe, (page 125) BBQ Sauce recipe, (page 122) and Sweet Zesty Mustard recipe, (page 132) are great condiments for this recipe. Just be sure to count the extra carbs.

3 servings @ 6.4 grams of usable carbs each.

Ham Patties

Servings: 4

3 cups Ham, ground, approximately 3/4 of a pound (0 carbs)
2 large Eggs
1/3 cup plain Pork Rinds, crushed fine
1 Tablespoon prepared Mustard (0 carbs)
2 Tablespoons Mayonnaise
2 Tablespoons Butter

Mix all ingredients, except butter, together in a medium bowl. Melt butter on medium heat in a large skillet until foaming subsides.

Shape mixture into 4 patties. Place in skillet and cook until browned, about 6 minutes. Turn and cook until browned on other side, about 7 minutes.

Note: Great with Sweet Zesty Mustard recipe, (page 132).

4 servings @ .6 grams of usable carbs each.

Pizza

Servings: 8

1 - recipe Pizza Crust (page 90)

Pizza Sauce:
3   Tablespoons Tomato Paste
1/2   cup Water
2   teaspoons bottled fresh minced Garlic or 4 cloves fresh Garlic, minced
1   teaspoon Fennel Seed
1   teaspoon Oregano Powder
1/4   teaspoon Salt

Toppings:
7   large Ripe Olives, sliced
5   fresh Mushrooms, wiped clean with damp paper towel and sliced or use canned Mushrooms
8   ounces Italian Sausage, broken up into pieces and browned until no pink remains
3   Tablespoons Onion, chopped
1/2   cup Parmesan Cheese, grated (I use DiGiorno® brand)
1/2   cup Cheddar Cheese, shredded
2   cups Mozzarella Cheese, shredded

Pizza Sauce
Mix all ingredients together in a small bowl. Spread evenly over crust.

Toppings
Spread toppings on evenly in order given.

Bake @ 425˚ for 10-12 minutes or until cheese is melted.

Note: I buy the 16 ounce frozen Italian Sausage rolls. Jimmy Dean® and Turkey Store® brands are low in carbs or you can use any brand that is low in carbs. Also, the Pizza Sauce can be used on any of your favorite recipes and it freezes very well.

8 servings of Pizza Sauce @ 1.2 grams of usable carbs each.

8 servings of Pizza Crust, Sauce, and Toppings @ 5.9 grams of usable carbs each.

Pizza Crust

Servings: 8

3/4 cup Warm Water
1   can Keto® Pizza Dough Mix
1   teaspoon Olive Oil
1   packet Yeast (included in dough mix)
1/4 teaspoon Garlic Powder
1/2 teaspoon Dried Basil Leaves
1   teaspoon Parmesan Cheese, grated (I use DiGiorno® brand)

Place all ingredients in bread machine in order given. Start machine on dough cycle. If too dry after a minute or so, add water a teaspoon at a time. If too wet, add parmesan cheese a teaspoon at a time. If your bread machine does not have a dough cycle use regular setting and remove dough after first kneading. If you do not have a bread machine, combine ingredients in a medium bowl and knead until smooth, about 10 minutes. Roll out to about a 14" circle or rectangle if you prefer. I roll it as thin as possible.

Pre-heat oven to 400°

Place on well oiled pizza pan or jelly roll pan. Bake for 10 minutes. Remove from oven and cool for 5 minutes before adding toppings.

Increase oven to 425°.

8 servings @ 2 grams of usable carbs each.

EAT YOURSELF THIN LIKE I DID!

Pork & Cabbage with Sauerkraut

Servings: 4

1 - 1 1/2 pound head of Cabbage, cut into 2" pieces
1/2 cup Water
1/2 teaspoon Salt
3 1/2 cups Pork Roast, cooked and coarsely chopped (leftover works fine)
2 cups Sauerkraut, drained
Sour Cream (optional)

Place cabbage and water in a large saucepan. Sprinkle with salt. Cook over medium-low heat until limp.

Add pork and sauerkraut, continue cooking until cabbage is done to your liking.

Serve immediately and pass Sour Cream at the table if desired.

Note: I like Vlasic® or Claussen® brand sauerkraut. Claussen® is found in the refrigerated section. Sour Cream is wonderful served with this dish, just be sure to count the extra carbs.

4 - 1 3/4 cup servings @ 4.2 grams of usable carbs each.

Pork Chops with Cream Gravy

Servings: 6

3 pounds Pork Chops
2 Tablespoons Cooking Oil
2 1/2 teaspoons Old Bay Seasoning® or your favorite seasoning
1/4 cup Water or Dry White Wine
3/4 cup Heavy Whipping Cream
1/4 teaspoon Xanthan Gum
Salt and Pepper to taste

Heat oil in a 12" skillet over medium-high heat until hot but not smoking. Brown pork chops in oil but don't over-crowd skillet. Brown in batches if necessary. Sprinkle with Old Bay Seasoning while browning.

When all are browned, reduce heat to lowest temperature and return all chops to skillet. Doesn't matter if they are layered at this point. Cover and cook 45 minutes or until tender. Check often and rearrange to cook evenly.

Remove chops to serving dish and cover with aluminum foil to keep warm.

Deglaze the pan with water or dry white wine on medium-high heat, scraping browned bits from bottom of pan. Add heavy whipping cream and salt and pepper to taste. Bring to a boil, SLOWLY sprinkle Xanthan Gum over, stirring briskly. Simmer for 1 minute or until thickened. Pour over pork chops and serve hot.

Note: Xanthan Gum is available in most health food stores and works great as a thickener. Just a little bit goes a long way.

6 servings @ 1 gram of usable carbs each.

Sweet & Sour Pork Vegetable Stir Fry

Servings: 4

2 Tablespoons Cooking Oil, preferably Peanut Oil

1 1/2 teaspoons bottled fresh minced Garlic or equivalent fresh Garlic, minced

1 teaspoon Chili Paste (found in Oriental food section) optional, this is hot

1/2 cup Onion, sliced lengthwise

1 medium Red or Green Bell Pepper, sliced in strips

8 ounces Zucchini, cut in half lengthwise and sliced into 1/4" half-rounds (about 2 - 2 1/2 cups)

8 ounce can Bamboo Shoots, drained, rinsed and drained again

4 cups Roast Pork Loin or Chops, cooked or leftover, cut in 1/4" strips

1 Tablespoon White Vinegar

3 Tablespoons Chicken or Beef Broth

2 teaspoons Fish Sauce (found in Oriental food section)

4 teaspoons Kikkoman® Soy Sauce

2 Tablespoons Splenda®, sugar substitute

1/4 teaspoon Xanthan Gum

In a small bowl mix together vinegar, broth, fish sauce, soy sauce, and Splenda.® Set aside.

Heat a large, heavy deep skillet or wok over medium-high heat for 1 minute. Add oil and swirl to cover bottom of pan and continue to heat for 1 minute. Add chili paste and garlic and stir fry for a few seconds. Add vegetables and stir fry for 2 minutes.

Add vinegar mixture. Then add pork and stir fry quickly to heat through. Stir in Xanthan Gum to thicken.

Serve immediately.

Note: If you don't like food with a little bite to it, you can omit the Chili Paste in this recipe for a mild flavored version.

4 servings @ 6.5 grams of usable carbs each.

Zucchini Boats

Servings: 6

3 medium Zucchini, washed, ends trimmed, and split in half lengthwise
1 - 12 ounce roll Jimmy Dean® 50% less fat Sausage
Garlic Powder to taste
Salt to taste
1/4 cup Water
1 cup Mozzarella Cheese, shredded
1 cup Cheddar Cheese, shredded

Pre-heat oven to 350°

Scoop seeds from Zucchini halves with a teaspoon and discard. Sprinkle scooped out cavities lightly with salt and garlic powder.

Divide sausage into 6 equal pieces and press into zucchini boats. Place in baking pan or large deep oven-proof skillet with lid. Pour water into bottom of pan and cover.

Bake @ 350° for 45 minutes. Remove from oven and top with cheddar and then mozzarella cheeses. Cover and return to oven for 5 minutes.

Note: If you like your foods a bit spicy, then sprinkle with some dried crushed red pepper. Also, great with Parmesan Cheese. Just remember to count the extra carbs.

6 servings @ 3.8 grams of usable carbs each.

Chicken Cacciatore

Servings: 3

1 1/2 pounds boneless, skinless Chicken Breasts and/or Thighs
2 Tablespoons Olive Oil
Salt and Pepper to taste
4 ounces fresh Mushrooms, sliced or 7 ounce can drained Mushrooms
1/2 cup Onion, sliced lengthwise
1 medium Red or Green Bell Pepper, seeds removed and sliced
    lengthwise
1 cup canned Tomatoes with juice, cut into pieces
1 Tablespoon Tomato Paste
1 Tablespoon bottled fresh minced Garlic or equivalent fresh Garlic,
    minced
1 teaspoon dried Oregano Leaves
1/2 teaspoon Fennel Seed (optional)
Pinch Crushed Red Pepper (optional)
2 Tablespoons Dry White Wine (optional)
1/2 cup Parmesan Cheese, grated (I use DiGiorno® brand)
1 cup Mozzarella Cheese, shredded

Brown chicken on both sides in hot olive oil, in a large skillet over medium heat.
Season with salt and pepper while browning. Remove chicken from pan. Reduce heat
and sauté onions and peppers until onions are soft, about 2 minutes. Add mushrooms
and sauté until limp, 2-3 minutes longer.

Add remaining ingredients except chicken, parmesan, and mozzarella cheeses. Bring to
a boil, reduce heat to simmer and add chicken pieces, spooning sauce over each piece.
Add small amount of water if too dry.

Simmer covered for 20-30 minutes or until chicken juice runs clear. Top each piece of
chicken with cheeses, replace cover until melted.

Serve hot.

Note: Sprinkle with crushed Red Pepper if you like it hot.

3 servings @ 10.9 grams of usable carbs each.

Chicken Olé

Servings: 4

2 pounds boneless, skinless Chicken Breasts and/or Thighs, cut into coarse chunks
1 Tablespoon Pure Olive Oil
Salt to taste
1/2 medium Red Bell Pepper, sliced into strips 1/4"x1" long
1/2 medium Green Bell Pepper, sliced into strips 1/4"x1" long
2 Tablespoons Onion, coarsely chopped
1 Tablespoon bottled fresh minced Garlic or equivalent fresh Garlic, minced
1 Tablespoon fresh squeezed Lime Juice
2 cups Cheddar Cheese, shredded

Heat olive oil in large, deep heavy non-stick skillet over medium-high heat until a haze forms. Brown chicken, sprinkle with salt, and turn to brown other side. Transfer chicken to a plate and set aside.

Reduce heat to medium-low, add onions and peppers to skillet and stir fry until tender crisp. Return chicken to pan and add garlic. Reduce heat to very low. Cover and cook 5-10 minutes or until chicken juices run clear. Watch closely so chicken doesn't burn.

Sprinkle with fresh lime juice and mix well. Spread evenly in pan and sprinkle with cheese. Cover and remove from heat.

Serve when cheese is melted.

Note: This recipe is a huge hit with everyone in my family and has become a signature recipe for my cooking shows and TV appearances. This is great served with Sour Cream, Salsa, and fresh Cilantro leaves. Just remember to count the extra carbs.

4 servings @ 4.4 grams of usable carbs each.

Chicken Parmigiana

Servings: 6

2 large Eggs
1 cup plain Pork Rinds, crushed fine
3/4 cup grated fresh Parmesan Cheese, divided (I use DiGiorno® brand)
2 Tablespoons Atkins® Bake Mix
3 Tablespoons Pure Olive Oil
2 Tablespoons Butter
3 pounds boneless, skinless Chicken Breasts (rinsed, dried, and pounded
    with a meat mallet or small heavy skillet between sheets of plastic
    wrap until 1/3" thick)
1 recipe Marinara Sauce, (page 124)
8 ounces Mozzarella Cheese, sliced

Beat eggs in a shallow dish and set aside.

Breading:

Mix pork rinds, 1/4 cup parmesan cheese, and bake mix in a shallow dish or pie pan. Set aside.

Pre-heat oven to 275°

Heat olive oil and butter in a large, non-stick skillet over medium-high heat until hot but do not let butter brown. When oil and butter are hot, dip chicken breasts in egg, then in breading, shaking off excess, and fry until well browned on each side. Do in batches if necessary. Place on large baking pan with sides and spread marinara sauce evenly over each piece.

Finish in oven for 10 minutes. Remove and top with remaining parmesan and mozzarella cheese. Return to oven for 5-8 minutes until cheese is melted. Serve immediately.

Note: Top with a little crushed Red Pepper if you like a little zing.

6 servings @ 4 grams of usable carbs each.

Quick Swiss Chicken & Broccoli Casserole

Servings: 6

1 medium head Broccoli Flowerets, washed or substitute frozen
1 Tablespoon Butter
2 cups fresh Mushrooms, sliced or 2 - 7 ounce cans, drained
1/4 cup Onion, chopped
3 cups cooked Chicken or Turkey, cut into coarse chunks or more if desired
2 large hard-cooked Eggs, sliced
4 ounces Swiss Cheese, shredded
3/4 cup Mayonnaise (0 carbs)
1/4 teaspoon Garlic Powder or 1/2 teaspoon if you prefer more Garlic flavor
Salt to taste

In a large, deep oven-proof skillet, cook broccoli in a small amount of salted boiling water, covered, just until tender-crisp. Drain and transfer to a medium bowl.

Pre-heat oven to 350°

Wipe out pan and melt butter in same pan over medium heat. Sauté onions until soft, about 3 minutes.

Add mushrooms and continue cooking until mushrooms are limp. Stir garlic powder into mayonnaise. Return broccoli to skillet along with chicken or turkey and mayonnaise. Toss gently until combined.

Top with hard-cooked egg slices then cheese. Cover and bake @ 350 for 30-40 minutes.

Serve immediately.

6 servings @ 4.5 grams of usable carbs each.

Sweet & Sour Chicken

Servings: 4

1 - recipe Sweet & Sour Sauce, (page 131)

1 1/2 pounds boneless, skinless Chicken Breasts, rinsed, dried, and cut
    into 1 1/2" pieces
2 large Egg Whites
1 cup plain Pork Rinds, crushed fine
1/4 cup Atkins® Bake Mix
1/2 teaspoon Garlic Powder
1/2 teaspoon Ground Ginger
Peanut Oil for frying

In a shallow dish, beat egg whites with a fork until foamy. Set aside.

Breading:
Mix pork rinds, bake mix, and spices in separate shallow dish. Set aside.

Heat oil in a deep fryer or heavy deep saucepan to 375° using a candy
thermometer. Dip chicken pieces in egg whites, then roll in breading, shaking
off excess.

Fry until nicely browned and cooked through, about 2-4 minutes each side.
Serve with Sweet & Sour Sauce recipe, (page 131).

Sweet & Sour Pork
Substitute equal amount of fresh uncooked pork, cut in chunks for the chicken
breasts. Proceed as directed.

Sweet & Sour Shrimp
Substitute equal amount of peeled and cleaned raw shrimp for the chicken.
Proceed as directed.

4 servings @ 4.6 grams of usable carbs each.

Broiled Halibut with Citrus Dill Butter

Servings: 2

1   pound Halibut Steaks
3   Tablespoons Butter, softened
1/2   teaspoon Lemon Zest, grated, yellow part only
1/2   teaspoon dried Dill Weed
Salt and Pepper to taste

Place Halibut on a broiler-safe pan. Mix remaining ingredients in a small bowl. Spread 1/3 of mixture on fish. Broil 5 inches from heat until fish is opaque and flakes easily with a fork. Do not over cook or Halibut will be dry. Time will vary depending on thickness of fish.

While fish is broiling, melt remaining butter mixture in a small saucepan and serve over Halibut. Salt and pepper to taste

Note: This is so delicious with my Tartar Sauce recipe, (page 133).

2 servings @ a trace of usable carbs each.

Crispy Fried Fish

Fish Fillets, your favorite kind, rinsed
1/4 cup Atkins® Bake Mix
1 teaspoon Cajun Seasoning or Seasoned Salt
1/2 cup Pork Rinds, crushed fine
1 large Egg
Peanut Oil

Pat fish dry with paper towels and set aside.

Breading:
Place bake mix, seasoning, and pork rinds in a shallow dish or pie plate and mix well. Set aside.

Beat egg in another shallow dish or pie plate. Heat oil 1/2" to 1" deep in large, heavy skillet (or use deep fryer) until hot but not smoking, temperature should be 375°. If using a heavy skillet, use candy thermometer for best results making sure the oil is back to correct temperature before adding next batch of fish.

Dip fillets in egg wash then dredge in breading, shaking off excess. Fry until brown and just opaque inside. Should flake easily with fork. Do not over cook or fish will be dry. Servings depend on amount of fish prepared.

Great served with my Tartar Sauce recipe, (page 133).

Note: This recipe works great whenever you are invited to a fish fry party. We just ask the hosts if they would save some fillets out for us and we bring our own breading. Just have the fillets damp before dredging into the breading mixture. We don't even bother with the egg wash at these parties.

Whole breading recipe and batter is 3.6 grams of usable carbs total.

Crusty Cajun Salmon with Cajun Mayonnaise

Servings: 2

1 pound Salmon Fillet
1 Tablespoon Butter, softened
4 Tablespoons Pork Rinds, crushed
3/4 teaspoon Cajun Seasoning

Cajun Mayonnaise:
3 Tablespoons Mayonnaise (0 carbs)
3/4 teaspoon Cajun Seasoning
1 teaspoon fresh Lime Juice (you can substitute Lemon Juice)

Pre-heat oven to 400°

Rinse Salmon and pat dry with paper towels. Place in shallow sprayed baking pan with sides. Spread butter over top.

Mix pork rinds and cajun seasoning and sprinkle over Salmon. Place in oven and bake @ 400° until Salmon flakes with a fork and is opaque. Do not over bake or Salmon will be dry. Time will vary depending on thickness of the fillet.

Cajun Mayonnaise
Stir all ingredients together in a small bowl and serve with Salmon.

Note: For a variation you can substitute Lemon Pepper for the Cajun Seasoning.

2 servings @ .9 grams of usable carbs each.

Greek Baked Salmon

Servings: 2

1 1/2 pounds Salmon Fillet, rinsed and patted dry with paper towels
1/4 cup Mayonnaise (0 carbs)
1/2 teaspoon Greek Seasoning (I use Cavenders® Greek Seasoning)
1 teaspoon fresh squeezed Lemon Juice
1/2 teaspoon Garlic Powder

Pre-heat oven to 375°

Place Salmon on a sprayed baking pan with sides. Mix remaining ingredients and spread evenly over Salmon.

Bake @ 375° for 25-30 minutes or until Salmon is opaque and flakes with a fork, depends on thickness of fillet. Do not over bake or it will be dry.

Note: This is one of my husband's favorite entrees.

2 servings @ 1.3 grams of usable carbs each.

Salmon Patties

Servings: 4

1 - 14.75 ounce can Salmon, drained, skinned, boned, and flaked
3 Tablespoons Green Onions, sliced (use green portion too)
2 Tablespoons Mayonnaise (0 carbs)
1 teaspoon dried Dill Weed
2 teaspoons fresh squeezed Lemon Juice (you can use thawed Minute
    Maid® Lemon Juice, not Lemonade)
1 large Egg
1/2 cup plain or spicy Pork Rinds, crushed fine
1/4 teaspoon Salt
1/8 teaspoon Pepper
3 Tablespoons Butter

Mix all ingredients together, except butter, in a medium bowl. Shape into 4 patties. Heat butter in a large skillet over medium heat until foaming subsides. Do not brown butter.

Add Salmon Patties and cook for about 3 minutes or until golden brown, then turn and cook about 3 minutes longer or until golden brown.

Note: Great with my Tartar Sauce recipe, (page 133).

4 servings @ 1.1 grams of usable carbs each.

Shrimp Scampi Parmesano

Servings: 2

1 pound Shrimp, raw fresh or thawed frozen, peeled and deveined
3 Tablespoons Butter
1 teaspoon bottled fresh minced Garlic or equivalent fresh Garlic,
    minced
1 teaspoon fresh squeezed Lemon Juice
2/3 cup Parmesan Cheese, shredded or grated
Salt to taste

Place shrimp in a sprayed baking pan with sides. Melt butter and mix with garlic and lemon juice. Pour over shrimp.

Salt lightly if desired. Broil shrimp just until shrimp turns pink and opaque. Watch closely, shrimp cooks fast.

Remove from broiler, sprinkle with cheese and return to broiler just until cheese melts.

Note: Serve with a lemon wedge or some Tartar Sauce recipe (page 133).

2 servings @ 2.2 grams of usable carbs each.

VEGETABLES

Baked "Potato" Casserole 107

Cauliflower Scramble 108

Creole Green Beans 109

Eggplant Parmigiana 110

Grilled Portabello Mushroom Caps 111

Ham & Swiss Green Beans 112

Italian Spinach 113

Marvelous Mushrooms 114

"Potato" Latke Pancakes 115

Sautéed Sesame Asparagus 116

Sweet & Spicy Red Cabbage 117

Zucchini Alfredo 118

Zucchini Italian Style 119

EAT YOURSELF THIN LIKE I DID!

Baked "Potato" Casserole

Servings: 4

3 cups Turnips, peeled and cut in 1" pieces, rinsed with water and
    drained
Salt to taste
2 ounces Cream Cheese, softened (4 Tablespoons)
1 Tablespoon Onion, chopped fine
2 Tablespoons Butter
1/2 cup Cheddar Cheese, shredded

Place turnips in medium sauce pan. Cover with water and add salt to taste.
Bring to a boil, reduce heat and cook covered until turnips are tender. Drain
well and mash or whip with an electric mixer.

Pre-heat oven to 350°

Add cream cheese, onion, butter, and mix well. Turn into a small buttered
casserole dish.

Bake @ 350° for about 35-40 minutes. Take out of oven and top with cheddar
cheese and return to oven approximately 5 minutes or until cheese is melted.

4 servings @ 4.8 grams of usable carbs each.

Cauliflower Scramble

Servings: 6

1 medium head Cauliflower, washed, trimmed and patted dry with paper towels
1 large Egg
2 Tablespoons Heavy Whipping Cream
2 Tablespoons Pure Olive Oil
3/4 teaspoon Salt
1 Tablespoon bottled fresh minced Garlic or equivalent fresh Garlic, minced

Cut cauliflower into flowerets and slice into 1/8" thick slices. Some will crumble and that's okay. Set aside. Beat egg and cream in a small bowl until blended and set aside.

Heat olive oil in a heavy large skillet over medium-high heat until a haze forms. Add cauliflower and salt. Make sure cauliflower is patted dry with paper towels or it will splatter.

Cook and stir cauliflower about 5 minutes until somewhat browned but still tender crisp. Stir in garlic and continue cooking and stirring about 1 minute.

Pour egg mixture over evenly and quickly stir to coat and cook until egg is set.

Serve immediately.

6 servings @ 3.2 grams of usable carbs each.

Creole Green Beans

Servings: 7

1 pound fresh or frozen Cut Green Beans, washed and trimmed
1/2 cup Water
4 strips Bacon
2 Tablespoons Onion, chopped
1/2 cup canned Tomatoes, cut up
Salt and Pepper to taste

Cook green beans in a medium saucepan with 1/2 cup salted water until desired doneness. Drain beans and set aside.

Fry bacon in a 10" skillet until crisp. Remove bacon from pan and drain on paper towels to remove excess grease. Pour off excess fat from skillet, and sauté onions until soft, about 2 minutes.

Crumble bacon into small pieces.

Add tomatoes, green beans, and bacon to onions and heat through.

Note: This recipe is not only quick and easy to make but it has also become a Holiday favorite with my family and works great for any occasion.

7 - 1/2 cup servings @ 2.2 grams of usable carbs each.

Eggplant Parmigiana

Servings: 12

2 medium Eggplants, about 1 pound each, washed and sliced into
   6 even slices, each
Salt
1 cup Pork Rinds, crushed fine
1/4 cup Atkins® Bake Mix
3 1/2 teaspoons dried Oregano Leaves, divided
3 teaspoons Garlic Powder, divided
3 large Egg Whites
4 Tablespoons Pure Olive Oil (use more if necessary)
1 cup Tomato Sauce (I use Hunts® brand)
1/2 teaspoon Fennel Seed (optional)
1 - 5.5 ounce can Tomato Juice (3/4 cup)
1/2 cup Parmesan Cheese, grated (I use DiGiorno® brand)
1 1/2 cups Mozzarella Cheese, shredded

Place eggplant in a colander in the sink and heavily sprinkle all surfaces with salt. Let set for 30 minutes. While eggplant is setting in colander, whisk together pork rinds, bake mix, 1 1/2 teaspoons oregano leaves, and 1 teaspoon garlic powder in a shallow dish. Set aside. In another shallow bowl beat egg whites with a fork until foamy. Set aside.

Pre-heat oven to 350°

Rinse eggplant slices and pat dry with paper towels. Heat olive oil in a large, heavy non-stick skillet over medium-high heat until a haze forms. Dip eggplant slices in egg whites, then into breading mixture, shaking off excess. Fry until browned, about 4 minutes per side. Don't over-crowd. Fry in batches if necessary. When browned, place pieces on a large, buttered, non-stick baking sheet with sides. You may need to use 2 baking sheets.

In a medium bowl whisk together tomato sauce, remaining 2 teaspoons oregano leaves, remaining 1 1/2 teaspoons garlic powder, 1/2 teaspoon fennel seed, and tomato juice. Pour evenly over eggplant.

Evenly sprinkle cheeses over top and bake in pre-heated oven @ 350° for 20 minutes or until eggplant is tender and cheese is melted.

Serve immediately.

12 servings @ 5.6 grams of usable carbs each.

EAT YOURSELF THIN LIKE I DID!

Grilled Portobello Mushroom Caps

Servings: 2

2 Portobello Mushroom Caps
1/4 cup Extra Virgin Olive Oil
1 Tablespoon Red Wine Vinegar
1/2 teaspoon Oregano Leaves
1 teaspoon bottled fresh minced Garlic or 2 Garlic cloves, minced
Salt to taste
1 Tablespoon fresh Parmesan Cheese, grated (I use DiGiorno® brand)

Mix all ingredients together, except mushroom caps and parmesan cheese. Place mushroom caps in quart size zip-top bag, pour marinade over and close. Distribute marinade to cover all surfaces. Redistribute every 15 minutes. Marinate 30-45 minutes.

Grill over medium coals or medium heat on gas grill for 2 1/2 minutes per side. Salt to taste. Sprinkle with parmesan cheese.

Serve immediately.

2 servings @ 2.5 grams of usable carbs each.

Ham & Swiss Green Beans

Servings: 5

1 pound fresh or frozen Cut Green Beans
1/2 cup Water
Salt to taste
1/2 cup Heavy Whipping Cream
1/4 cup Water
3/4 cup Ham, cut into 1/4" dice (0 carbs)
2 ounces Swiss Cheese, cut in small cubes
1/4 teaspoon Garlic Powder
1/2 teaspoon Xanthan Gum

Bring 1/2 cup salted water to a boil in a 3 quart saucepan. Add green beans, bring to a boil again. Cover, reduce heat and cook until desired doneness. Drain and discard liquid. Place into a serving bowl and cover with foil to keep warm.

Pour heavy whipping cream and water into the same saucepan and heat over medium heat until hot but not boiling. Add remaining ingredients, except Xanthan Gum, and stir until cheese is melted. Sprinkle Xanthan Gum slowly over sauce and whisk well until thickened. Return green beans to sauce and heat through.

Note: Xanthan Gum is a great thickener and can be found in most health food stores. Remember that just a tiny bit goes a long way.

5 servings @ 3.4 grams of usable carbs each.

Italian Spinach

Servings: 4

10 ounces fresh Spinach, pre-washed package
2 Tablespoons Pure Olive Oil
3 large cloves Garlic, minced or equivalent bottled fresh minced Garlic
2 Tablespoons Onion, chopped
1/2 teaspoon dried Basil Leaves
1/2 teaspoon Salt
1/4 cup Parmesan Cheese, grated (I use DiGiorno® brand)
Pepper to taste

Sauté onion in olive oil in large skillet over medium heat until soft but not browned. Add garlic, basil, spinach, salt, and pepper.

Cook covered over low heat until very limp. Remove cover and cook until most of liquid is evaporated.

Divide into 4 servings and sprinkle each with 1 Tablespoon of parmesan cheese.

Serve immediately.

4 servings @ 1.5 grams of usable carbs each.

Marvelous Mushrooms

Servings: 3

1 Tablespoon Butter
8 ounces fresh Mushrooms, wiped clean and sliced
1 teaspoon Greek Seasoning (I use Cavenders® brand)
1 teaspoon bottled fresh minced Garlic or 2 small Garlic cloves, minced
1/4 cup Dry White Wine
Salt to taste

Melt butter over medium heat in a small saucepan. Add mushrooms and sauté stirring frequently until mushrooms are limp. Stir in remaining ingredients, except salt, and bring to a boil over medium-high heat.

Boil, stirring frequently until most liquid is evaporated. Add salt to taste.

Note: This is delicious served on your favorite steak and is especially wonderful on Prime Rib. Quick and easy and refrigerates very well.

3 servings @ 2.3 grams of usable carbs each.

"Potato" Latke Pancakes

Servings: 5

2 1/2 cups Daikon Radish or Turnip, peeled and shredded (look in
    produce section near Oriental vegetables for Daikon Radish, large,
    long, and cream colored)
1 large Egg
2 Tablespoons Onion, chopped fine
1 Tablespoon Atkins® Bake Mix
1/2 teaspoon Salt
Butter for frying

Mix all ingredients together in a medium bowl, except butter. Heat butter in a
large non-stick skillet over medium heat until foaming subsides. Drop by
spoonfuls to make 5 pancakes using the back of a spoon to spread thin.

Cook over medium heat until underside is browned. Turn and cook until well
browned and cooked through.

Note: Try one of these delicious accompaniments -

1 Tablespoon unsweetened Applesauce @ 1.5 grams of carbs.

1 strip crisp fried Bacon @ 0 grams of carbs.

1 Tablespoon Sour Cream @ .5 grams of carbs.

5 servings @ 2.5 grams of usable carbs each using Daikon Radish.

5 servings @ 3.5 grams of usable carbs each using Turnips.

Sautéed Sesame Asparagus

Servings: 3

2 Tablespoons Cooking Oil
1 pound fresh Asparagus, washed well, tough ends snapped off, dried
     and cut in 1 1/2" pieces diagonally
1/2 teaspoon Salt
2 teaspoons Kikkoman® Soy Sauce
1 teaspoon Toasted Sesame Oil

Heat cooking oil in large, heavy non-stick skillet over medium-high heat until hot but not smoking. Add asparagus, sprinkle with salt, and sauté until tender crisp.

Sprinkle with soy sauce and sesame oil and serve immediately.

3 servings @ 3 grams of usable carbs each.

Sweet & Spicy Red Cabbage

Servings: 20

4 strips Bacon
1 - 1 3/4 pound head of Red Cabbage, shredded
1 cup Water
5 Tablespoons Red Wine Vinegar
3 Tablespoons Brown Sugar Twin®, sugar substitute
1/8 teaspoon Ground Allspice
1/8 teaspoon Ground Cloves
1 teaspoon Salt
Pepper to taste

Fry bacon in large deep skillet over low heat, turning frequently until crisp. Remove bacon and set aside. Crumble when cool.

Add all remaining ingredients, except red cabbage, to bacon drippings. Mix well and add red cabbage and bacon.

Stir until combined. Cover and cook over low heat until red cabbage is soft, approximately 20-30 minutes.

Note: Keeps well in refrigerator and it reheats very well.

20 - 1/2 cup servings @ 1.5 grams of usable carbs each.

Zucchini Alfredo

Servings: 4

2 Tablespoons Pure Olive Oil
2 large Zucchini, sliced 1/4" thick (about 2 pounds)
1 1/2 teaspoons Salt, divided
2 teaspoons bottled fresh minced Garlic or equivalent fresh Garlic, minced
1/2 cup Heavy Whipping Cream
1 cup Parmesan Cheese, shredded (I use DiGiorno® brand)

Heat olive oil in large non-stick skillet over medium-high heat. Add zucchini, sprinkle with salt, and stir fry for 3 minutes.

Add heavy whipping cream and garlic. Mix gently.

Sprinkle with parmesan cheese, turn heat off and cover until cheese is melted.

Serve immediately.

Note: We enjoy a little crushed Red Pepper sprinkled over the top.

4 servings @ 5.1 grams of usable carbs each.

Zucchini Italian Style

Servings: 6

4 medium Zucchini, washed and sliced 1/4" thick (2 1/2 pounds)
1/2 cup canned Tomatoes, chopped
1 Tablespoon Tomato Paste
1/2 teaspoon bottled fresh minced Garlic or equivalent fresh Garlic, minced
1/2 teaspoon Salt
1/2 teaspoon dried Oregano Leaves
1/2 teaspoon dried Basil Leaves
1/4 teaspoon Fennel Seed
1/2 cup Parmesan Cheese, shredded (I use DiGiorno® brand)
1/2 cup Mozzarella Cheese, shredded

Pre-heat oven to 350°

Toss all ingredients, except cheeses, together in a large bowl. Transfer to a sprayed baking dish sufficient size to hold. Cover with aluminum foil and bake @ 350° for 20-25 minutes.

Remove foil, sprinkle with parmesan and mozzarella cheeses, return to oven for an additional 10 minutes. Remove from oven and let stand 5 minutes.

Serve immediately.

6 servings @ 4.1 grams of usable carbs each.

SAUCES & CONDIMENTS

Alfredo Sauce. 121

BBQ Sauce. 122

Berry Sauce 123

Marinara Sauce 124

Nancy's Ketchup 125

Nancy's Pico De Gallo 126

Nancy's Steak Sauce 127

Nancy's Strawberry Spread 128

Nancy's Maple Butter 128

Sweet Vanilla Butter 128

Pesto Cream Sauce 129

Spicy Seafood Cocktail Sauce 130

Sweet & Sour Sauce 131

Sweet Zesty Mustard Sauce 132

Nancy's Tartar Sauce 133

EAT YOURSELF THIN LIKE I DID!

Alfredo Sauce

Servings: 7

3 Tablespoons Butter
1 1/2 cups Heavy Whipping Cream
1/2 cup fresh Parmesan Cheese, grated (I use DiGiorno® brand)
1/4 teaspoon Salt
1 teaspoon bottled fresh minced Garlic or equivalent fresh Garlic, minced

Melt butter in a small saucepan over low heat. Add heavy whipping cream and stir. Add parmesan cheese, salt, and garlic and stir until heated through. Do not boil. Makes 1 3/4 cups.

Serve immediately.

Note: This is delicious served over Grilled Chicken, Steamed Vegetables, or even Stuffed Mushrooms and it's also quick and easy.

7 - 1/4 cup servings @ 1.7 grams of usable carbs each.

BBQ Sauce

Servings: 22

1 - 6 ounce can Tomato Paste
1 cup Water
2 Tablespoons White Vinegar
2 1/2 Tablespoons Brown Sugar Twin®, sugar substitute
1 Tablespoon bottled fresh minced Garlic or equivalent fresh Garlic, minced
1/4 teaspoon Liquid Smoke flavoring (1/2 teaspoon if you like a real smoky flavor)
1/4 teaspoon Salt
1 teaspoon Worcestershire Sauce
Tabasco Sauce to taste (optional)

Place tomato paste in a medium, heavy saucepan. Gradually add water, stirring well with each addition to smooth out lumps.

Stir in remaining ingredients and simmer on low heat for about 15 minutes.

Store in refrigerator.

Note: Great on your favorite meats like Ribs, Burgers, Steaks, Pork Chops, or Chicken.

22 - 1 Tablespoon servings @ 1.4 grams of usable carbs each.

Berry Sauce

1   pint fresh Berries
2   Tablespoons Splenda®, sugar substitute
1/4   teaspoon liquid Sweet'N Low®, sugar substitute

Wash berries, except strawberries, (see directions below for strawberry sauce) and place in a small saucepan. Add Splenda and liquid Sweet'N Low. Do not add water, the water clinging to the berries is sufficient.

Cook over low heat, stirring frequently. Cook until syrupy and slightly thickened. If not sweet enough, add more liquid Sweet'N Low. It will not add more carbs.

Chill in refrigerator, covered.

Strawberry Sauce:
Wash, hull, and slice Strawberries, then toss with 2 Tablespoons of Splenda and 1/2 teaspoon liquid Sweet'N Low, mashing slightly. Let stand for 20 minutes, then refrigerate, covered until serving time.

Note: These recipes are fabulous over Cheesecake.

Blackberries -
1 pint = 3/4 cup finished sauce - 12 Tablespoons @ 1.9 grams of usable carbs
    each.

Blueberries -
1 pint = 3/4 cup finished sauce - 12 Tablespoons @ 4 grams of usable carbs
    each.

Raspberries -
1 pint = 1 1/3 cups finished sauce - 21 Tablespoons @ .8 grams of usable carbs
    each.

Strawberries -
1 pint = 2 cups finished sauce - 32 Tablespoons @ .6 grams usable carbs each.

Marinara Sauce

Servings: 5

1 Tablespoon Pure Olive Oil
2 Tablespoons Onion, chopped fine
2 teaspoons bottled fresh minced Garlic or equivalent fresh Garlic, minced
1 - 5.5 ounce can of Tomato Juice (3/4 cup)
1 Tablespoon Tomato Paste
1/4 teaspoon Salt
1/8 teaspoon Pepper
1/4 teaspoon Splenda®, sugar substitute
1/4 teaspoon dried Basil Leaves
1/4 teaspoon dried Oregano Leaves
1/8 teaspoon Fennel Seed
Pinch of dried crushed Red Pepper (optional)

Heat olive oil in a small saucepan over medium heat until a haze appears. Add onion and sauté for about 2 minutes until soft. Do not brown.

Add garlic and cook for 1 minute. Add remaining ingredients and mix well. Simmer for about 15 minutes over low heat.

Whole recipe has only 12.5 grams of usable carbs total.

Note: Wonderful served over steamed shredded Zucchini, Meatballs, or Grilled Chicken Breasts.

5 - 3 Tablespoon servings @ 2.5 grams of usable carbs each.

Nancy's Ketchup

Servings: 32

1 - 6 ounce can Tomato Paste
2 Tablespoons White Vinegar
3 Tablespoons Splenda®, sugar substitute or (1 1/2 teaspoons liquid
   Sweet'N Low®, sugar substitute)
1/2 teaspoon Garlic Powder
1/2 teaspoon Onion Juice (I use McCormick® brand)
Pinch of Allspice
Pinch of Salt
1 1/4 cups Water

Mix all ingredients, except water, together in a small saucepan. Add water a little at a time to smooth out lumps. Cook over low heat for 15 minutes to blend flavors.

Chill and store in refrigerator. Keeps well.

Note: I put my Ketchup in a squeeze bottle to make it quick and easy to dispense. Shake well before using.

32 Tablespoon servings @ .8 grams of usable carbs each using liquid Sweet'N Low®.

32 Tablespoon servings @ 1 gram of usable carbs each using Splenda®.

Nancy's Pico De Gallo
Servings: 13

2   cups Tomatoes, cored, seeded and chopped into 1/4" dice
    (Roma Tomatoes work best)
1   cup Onion, chopped
1   teaspoon bottled fresh minced Garlic or equivalent fresh Garlic,
    minced
1/2 fresh Jalapeño Pepper, seeded and minced fine
1/2 teaspoon Salt
1/4 cup fresh Cilantro Leaves, whole (in produce section near the
    Parsley)
2   Tablespoons Cooking Oil
2   teaspoons Lime Juice

Mix all ingredients together in a medium bowl.

Cover and refrigerate to blend flavors. Stays fresh 1 day.

Note: You can adjust the amount of Jalapeño Pepper to your taste. Most are fairly mild once you seed them. This recipe is great with my Chicken Olé recipe, (page 96) or use for dipping Pork Rinds.

13 - 1/4 cup servings @ 3.2 grams of usable carbs each.

Nancy's Steak Sauce

Servings: 22

2/3 cup Hunts® Tomato Sauce
1 Tablespoon Brown Sugar Twin®, sugar substitute
1/4 teaspoon Dry Mustard
1/2 teaspoon Turmeric Powder
1/2 teaspoon Garlic Powder
1 teaspoon Onion Juice (I use McCormick® brand)
1 teaspoon Cooking Oil
2 teaspoons Worcestershire Sauce (0 carbs)
1/4 cup Water
1/2 teaspoon White Vinegar

In a small saucepan mix all ingredients well and simmer over low heat for 15 minutes.

Makes 1 1/4 cups total.

Store in refrigerator. Keeps very well.

Note: Using a squeeze bottle sure makes serving quick and easy. Shake well before using.

22 - 1 Tablespoon servings @ .4 grams of usable carbs each.

Nancy's Strawberry Spread

Servings: 10

2 Tablespoons Butter, softened
2 ounces Cream Cheese, softened
2 Tablespoons Heavy Whipping Cream
3 Tablespoons Splenda®, sugar substitute, divided
1/4 cup Strawberries, diced

Stir 1 Tablespoon of Splenda® into strawberries in small bowl and set aside. Mix remaining ingredients in small bowl, add strawberries and mix well.

Cover and refrigerate.

Note: Delicious served on Strawberry Walnut Muffins, (page 32).

10 - 1 Tablespoon servings @ .9 grams of usable carbs each.

Sweet Vanilla Butter
4 Tablespoons Butter, softened
2 1/2 teaspoons Splenda®, sugar substitute
1/2 teaspoon Vanilla Extract

Mix all together in small bowl. Turn out onto plastic wrap and form into log, using plastic wrap to assist. Store in refrigerator. Slice off rounds as needed. Be sure to slice into 12 equal rounds.

Note: Great on Sour Cream Poppyseed Muffins, (page 30).

12 slices @ .2 grams of usable carbs each.

Nancy's Maple Butter
Substitute 1/2 teaspoon Maple Flavored Extract for Vanilla Extract.

Note: Maple Butter is terrific on Butterscotch Pecan Muffins, (page 26).

12 slices @ .2 grams of usable carbs each.

Pesto Cream Sauce

Servings: 6

3/4 cup Heavy Whipping Cream
1/4 cup Water
2 Tablespoons Butter
1/4 cup prepared Pesto Sauce (found in refrigerated area in produce section)
1 teaspoon bottled fresh minced Garlic or equivalent fresh Garlic, minced
1/4 teaspoon Salt
3/4 cup Parmesan Cheese, shredded and divided (I use DiGiorno® brand)

Heat heavy whipping cream and water in a small, heavy saucepan over medium heat until hot but not boiling. Add butter, pesto sauce, garlic, and salt. Reduce heat and continue to cook about 5 more minutes over low heat.

Stir in 1/2 cup parmesan cheese until melted. Use remaining parmesan cheese to sprinkle over top.

Serve immediately.

Note: This is one of those recipes your guests will rave about. They'll think you spent all day when it's actually quick and easy. Wonderful served over grilled meats or vegetables.

6 servings @ 1.7 grams of usable carbs each.

Spicy Seafood Cocktail Sauce

Servings: 9

1/2 cup Nancy's Ketchup recipe, (page 125) or equivalent low carb
  Ketchup
1 Tablespoon prepared Horseradish
1/2 teaspoon Worcestershire Sauce
1 teaspoon fresh squeezed Lemon Juice

Combine all ingredients in a small bowl.

Cover and refrigerate.

Note: Serve with any of your favorite seafood recipes. Great for Shrimp Cocktail.

Makes 9 1/2 Tablespoons.

1 Tablespoon serving @ .9 grams of usable carbs.

Sweet & Sour Sauce

Servings: 4

1 1/2 cups Chicken Broth (0 carbs)
1/4 cup White Vinegar
1/4 cup Splenda®, sugar substitute
1 teaspoon bottled fresh minced Garlic or equivalent fresh Garlic, minced
1/4 cup Nancy's Ketchup recipe, (page 125) or equivalent low carb Ketchup
1 teaspoon Cooking Oil
1 teaspoon Xanthan Gum
1/4 medium Onion, cut in 1" squares
1/8 medium Red Bell Pepper, cut into 1" squares
1/8 medium Green Bell Pepper, cut into 1" squares

Mix first 6 ingredients together in a small saucepan. Bring to a boil and sprinkle Xanthan gum in gradually, whisking constantly. Simmer until thickened.

Add peppers and onions and reduce heat to keep warm.

Note: Xanthan Gum works great as a thickener and can be found at most health food stores. Serve over Sweet & Sour Chicken, Pork, or Shrimp recipes, (page 99). Great on Grilled Chicken or Fish.

4 servings @ 3.8 grams of usable carbs each.

Sweet Zesty Mustard Sauce

Servings: 10

1/2 cup prepared Yellow Mustard
2 Tablespoons Brown Sugar Twin®, sugar substitute
2 Tablespoons Nancy's Ketchup recipe, (page 125) or equivalent low
   carb Ketchup
1 teaspoon prepared Horseradish
1/4 teaspoon Ground Cloves

Mix all ingredients together.

Keep covered and refrigerated. Always shake or stir well before using.

Note: I like to store this recipe in a squeeze bottle making it quick and easy to use. Makes an excellent glaze for ham. One recipe makes enough for a large bone-in half ham with enough left to serve as a condiment. Also, great with burgers and hot dogs.

10 servings @ .5 grams of usable carbs each.

Nancy's Tartar Sauce

Servings: 34

1 cup Mayonnaise (0 carbs)
1 Tablespoon Onion, grated with juice
2 Tablespoons Dill Pickle, grated
3 Tablespoons Parsley, chopped fine
1 Tablespoon fresh squeezed Lemon Juice

Place all ingredients in a medium bowl and mix well.

Store covered and refrigerated.

Note: My Tartar Sauce recipe has been so well received that even a 5 Star restaurant in Lakeville, Minnesota uses it. Delicious on all of your favorite Seafood recipes, I hope your family and friends will love it.

34 - 1 Tablespoon servings @ only a trace of usable carbs each.

DESSERTS

Blueberry Dream Squares 135
Boston Cream Pie 136
Butterscotch Pecan Cheesecake 137
Cherry Cinnamon Dessert 138
Cherry Swirl 139
Chinese Almond Cookies. 140
Chocolate Almond Ice Cream. 141
Chocolate Cheesecake. 142
Chocolate Cupcakes 143
Chocolate Cream Frosting 144
Chocolate Glaze 145
Crust For Pie. 146
Dessert Crust 146
Sweetened Whipped Cream. 147
Frozen Whipped Cream Clouds. 147
Lemon Cheesecake 148
Orange Cheesecake. 148
Lime Cheesecake. 148
Lemon Meringue Pie 149
Lime Frosted Jell-O 150
Old-Fashioned Vanilla Pudding 151
Chocolate Pudding. 151
Peanut Butter & Chocolate Patties 152
Pistachio Ice Cream. 153
Pumpkin Pecan Dessert 154
Strawberry Cheesecake. 155
Strawberry Crepes 156
Strawberry-Kiwi Puff 157
Strawberry Snowballs. 158

Blueberry Dream Squares

Servings: 12

1 - recipe Dessert Crust, (page 146) prepare and let cool completely

Filling:
2 - 8 ounce packages Cream Cheese, softened
1/4 cup Splenda®, sugar substitute
1/4 teaspoon liquid Sweet'N Low®, sugar substitute
1 teaspoon Vanilla Extract
1 cup Heavy Whipping Cream (whipped until thick but not stiff)
1 teaspoon sugar-free Jell-O® instant Vanilla pudding mix

Berry Layer:
3/4 cup fresh or frozen Blueberries
2 Tablespoons Splenda®, sugar substitute

Topping:
1 cup Heavy Whipping Cream
1 Tablespoon sugar-free Jell-O® instant Vanilla pudding mix
1 teaspoon Vanilla Extract

Filling: Whip cream cheese with an electric mixer until smooth and fluffy. Add Splenda®, liquid Sweet'N Low®, and vanilla extract. Whip until blended. Set aside. Sprinkle pudding mix over whipped cream in medium bowl and stir in. Fold whipped cream into cream cheese mixture and spread evenly over crust. Make sure the crust is cooled first. Chill.

Berry Layer: In a small saucepan mix blueberries and Splenda® together and cook over low heat until syrupy. Cool completely, then spoon berry mixture over filling. Chill while making topping.

Topping: Mix Topping ingredients together and whip with electric mixer until very thick but not too stiff. Spread over berries. Refrigerate covered.

Note: This is a huge hit with my family and especially my husband.

12 servings @ 8.3 grams of usable carbs each.

Boston Cream Pie

Servings: 6

1 - recipe Old-Fashioned Vanilla Pudding, (page 151) make ahead and
   chill
1 - recipe Chocolate Glaze, (page 145) make ahead and chill

Batter:
1/2 cup Atkins® Bake Mix
1 teaspoon Guar Gum
1 teaspoon Baking Powder
4 Tablespoons Splenda®, sugar substitute
1 cup Heavy Whipping Cream
1/2 cup Water
4 large Eggs
2 teaspoons Vanilla Extract
1/2 teaspoon Almond Extract

Pre-heat oven to 350°

Whisk bake mix, Guar Gum, baking powder, and Splenda® together in medium bowl.
Add remaining ingredients and whisk batter until smooth.

Divide evenly into 2 well buttered, non-stick 8" round cake pans. I also line the bottom
with parchment paper. Bake @ 350° for 22-25 minutes, until lightly browned and
middle springs back when touched with finger.

Cool in pans on racks for 5 minutes. Turn out of pans and finish cooling on racks. Wrap
with plastic wrap when completely cooled. Store in refrigerator until ready to assemble.

Assembly: Place 1 cake layer upside down on cake plate. Spread vanilla pudding over
top. Place second cake layer right side up over pudding layer. Pour chocolate glaze over
top and spread to run down sides. Chill until serving time. Refrigerate leftovers.

Note: Cakes can be made a day ahead and wrapped in plastic and
   refrigerated. Assemble 1 or 2 hours before serving. Guar Gum works great
   as a thickener and can be found in most health food stores.

6 servings @ 7.4 grams of usable carbs each.

Butterscotch Pecan Cheesecake

Servings: 16

Butter for greasing pan
1/2 cup Pecans, toasted, finely chopped, and divided
1 Tablespoon Brown Sugar Twin®, sugar substitute
5 - 8 ounce packages Cream Cheese, softened
1/4 pound Butter, softened (1 stick)
1 cup Heavy Whipping Cream
1 Tablespoon Vanilla Extract
2/3 cup Splenda®, sugar substitute
1 small package sugar-free Jell-O® instant Butterscotch pudding mix
6 large Eggs, yolks broken

Pre-heat oven to 325°

Grease sides and bottom of 9 springform pan heavily with butter. I also line the bottom with parchment paper, then butter. Sprinkle 1/4 cup of pecans evenly on bottom, then sprinkle with 1 Tablespoon of Brown Sugar Twin®. Cover outside bottom and sides with doubled foil to keep from leaking. Set aside.

Whip cream cheese and butter in a large mixing bowl with an electric mixer until smooth and creamy. Set aside.

In a medium mixing bowl whisk heavy whipping cream, vanilla extract, Splenda®, and butterscotch pudding mix. Mixture will become very stiff. Add to cream cheese, 1/4 at a time, beating until smooth with each addition. Add eggs all at once on low speed, just until incorporated. DO NOT OVERMIX or cheesecake will be grainy instead of creamy.

Pour into prepared pan and rap on countertop a few times to release air bubbles. Sprinkle remaining pecans on top.

Bake @ 325° for 60-70 minutes or until just set. Turn off oven and leave in for 1 additional hour. Take out and finish cooling at room temperature. Do not remove sides of pan until completely cooled to room temperature. Cover and refrigerate at least 6 hours before serving. Keep refrigerated. Cheesecake will get firmer as it chills.

16 servings @ 5.2 grams of usable carbs each.

Cherry Cinnamon Dessert

Servings: 9

2 small packages sugar-free Cherry Jell-O®
1 1/2 cups Boiling Water
2 cups Cold Water
1/2 cup unsweetened Applesauce (1 single serving size small plastic
     container)
1 teaspoon Ground Cinnamon and extra for garnish

1 - recipe Sweetened Whipped Cream, (page 147)

Dissolve Jell-O® in boiling water in a 9" square or 7"x11" pan. Stir well until fully dissolved. This takes at least 2 minutes.

Stir in cold water and refrigerate until syrupy. Mix cinnamon into applesauce then add to Jell-O®, mixing well.

Refrigerate until firm. Spread sweetened whipped cream over top and lightly sprinkle with cinnamon.

Serve and enjoy.

9 servings @ 2.4 grams of usable carbs each.

Cherry Swirl
Servings: 12

Jell-O:
2 small packages sugar-free Cherry Jell-O®
1 cup Boiling Water
3 cups Cold Water

Cream Cheese Swirl:
4 ounces Cream Cheese, softened
3/4 cup Heavy Whipping Cream
1/2 cup Water
2 Tablespoons sugar-free Jell-O® instant Vanilla pudding mix
1 teaspoon Vanilla Extract
4 Tablespoons Splenda®, sugar substitute

Jell-O: Stir boiling water into Jell-O® in a medium bowl until completely dissolved. Stir in cold water and refrigerate.

Cream Cheese Swirl: Whip cream cheese in a medium bowl until very smooth and fluffy. Set aside. Measure heavy whipping cream into a

2 cup glass measuring cup or bowl. Add vanilla pudding mix, vanilla extract, and Splenda®. Whisk until smooth. Whisk pudding mixture gradually into cream cheese. Whisk in water. Set aside until Jell-O® is syrupy. Do not let Jell-O® set up.

Pour Jell-O® into a 7"x11" pan. Drop cream cheese mixture by spoonfuls over Jell-O® and swirl by cutting through, back and forth with a knife. Refrigerate until set.

Note: A delicious option is to add 1/2 cup canned, drained, sour pie cherries, no sugar added, packed in water, and 2 Tablespoons Splenda to Jell-O® when syrupy. Continue as directed. Measure and freeze leftover cherries in a lock-top freezer bag.

12 servings @ 2.2 grams of usable carbs each without cherries.

12 servings @ 3.1 grams of usable carbs each with cherries.

Chinese Almond Cookies

Servings: 20

1/4 pound Butter, softened (1 stick)
1 Tablespoon Peanut Butter or low carb Peanut Butter (no more than 6 grams of carbs per 2 Tablespoons)
1 large Egg
1/2 cup Splenda®, sugar substitute
1 teaspoon Almond Extract
1/2 teaspoon Baking Powder
1/8 teaspoon Salt
1/4 cup Atkins® Bake Mix
1/4 cup Blanched Almond Flour
1/4 cup sliced Almonds, toasted

Pre-heat oven to 350°

In a medium mixing bowl, cream butter and peanut butter together.

Add egg, Splenda®, almond extract, baking powder, and salt. Mix well. Stir in bake mix, almond flour, and sliced almonds.

Drop from a spoon onto a buttered cookie sheet, shaping nicely with a spoon. Bake @ 350° for about 10 minutes or until lightly browned. Let cookie sheet cool between batches or cookies will spread too much.

Note: Store loosely covered. Serve cold or warm.

20 servings @ 1 gram of usable carbs each.

Chocolate Almond Ice Cream

Servings: 12

2 1/2 cups plus 2 Tablespoons Heavy Whipping Cream, divided
12 ounces Cream Cheese, softened (1 1/2 - 8 ounce packages)
3 Tablespoons Butter, softened
3/4 cup Splenda®, sugar substitute
1 1/2 teaspoons Vanilla Extract
1/8 teaspoon Salt
1/2 cup plus 1 Tablespoon Water
1/4 cup sliced Almonds, toasted
1 large package sugar-free Jell-O® instant Chocolate pudding mix
   (6 servings)

Whip 1 1/2 cups of heavy whipping cream with electric mixer in medium bowl until thick. Do not over beat. Set aside. Place cream cheese in large bowl and whip on high with same beaters until smooth and fluffy.

Mix in all remaining ingredients, except chocolate pudding mix and whipped cream, along with remaining unwhipped heavy whipping cream. Mix until just combined and smooth. Add chocolate pudding mix and whipped cream and mix on low speed until smooth.

Pour into 9"x5"x2 3/4" bread pan. Will be quite full or you can pour into 12 paper cups. Cover with plastic wrap.

Place in freezer until frozen all the way through. Usually takes overnight. Slice into 12 equal servings and cover leftovers. Or freeze in an electric ice cream freezer.

Note: Place in microwave on low for 15 seconds to soften.

12 servings @ 7.5 grams of usable carbs each.

Chocolate Cheesecake
Servings: 16

5 - 8 ounce packages Cream Cheese, softened
1/4 pound Butter, softened (1 stick)
1 cup Heavy Whipping Cream
2 teaspoons Vanilla Extract
3/4 cup Splenda®, sugar substitute
2 - 1 ounce squares unsweetened Baking Chocolate, melted
1 - 1.4 ounce package sugar-free Jell-O® instant Chocolate pudding mix
6 large Eggs, yolks broken

Pre-heat oven to 325°

Whip cream cheese and butter in a large mixing bowl with an electric mixer until smooth and fluffy. Set aside. In a medium mixing bowl, whisk heavy whipping cream, vanilla extract, Splenda®, melted chocolate, and chocolate pudding mix. Mixture will become very stiff. Add to cream cheese, 1/4 at a time and whip until smooth.

When all is smooth, add eggs all at once. Mix on low speed just until eggs are incorporated. Do not over mix or texture will be grainy instead of creamy.

Spray a 9" springform pan, I also line the bottom with parchment paper, and cover the outside bottom and sides with doubled aluminum foil to prevent leakage. Pour mixture into pan and rap on countertop a few times to release air bubbles.

Bake @ 325° for 60-70 minutes or until just set. Turn off oven and leave in 1 additional hour. Finish cooling at room temperature. Do not remove sides of pan until completely cooled to room temperature. Cover and refrigerate at least 6 hours. Cheesecake will get firmer as it chills.

Note: This one is a family favorite for "Chocolate Lovers".

16 servings @ 5.5 grams of usable carbs each.

Chocolate Cupcakes

Servings: 18

4 large Eggs, separated
3/4 teaspoon Cream of Tartar
1 - 2.1 ounce package sugar-free Jell-O® instant Chocolate pudding mix
(6 serving size), divided. Save remaining pudding mix for frosting,
   (page 144)
1/2 cup Heavy Whipping Cream
1/2 cup Water
1/2 cup Splenda®, sugar substitute
1 teaspoon Baking Powder
1 teaspoon Vanilla Extract

Pre-heat oven to 350°

Place egg whites and cream of tartar in a medium mixing bowl and set aside.
Measure 6 Tablespoons of pudding mix and set aside. Mix egg yolks, heavy
whipping cream and water in a large bowl. Add Splenda®, baking powder,
vanilla extract, and the 6 Tablespoons of pudding mix and whisk until smooth.
Set aside.

Whip egg whites and cream of tartar with an electric mixer until stiff but not
dry. Gently fold chocolate mixture into egg whites. Divide evenly into 18
buttered, non-stick mini-muffin pans.

Bake @ 350° for 18-20 minutes. Cool in pans. They will fall, this is the nature
of this mixture.

When cool frost with Chocolate Cream Frosting recipe, (page 144).

Note: Best served cold. For a real treat, store these frosted cupcakes in the
   freezer and eat them frozen. They taste like a candy bar.

18 servings @ 3 grams of usable carbs each without frosting.

18 servings @ 4.5 grams of usable carbs each with frosting.

Chocolate Cream Frosting

Servings: 18

4 ounces Cream Cheese, softened
1 Tablespoon Butter, softened
6 Tablespoons Heavy Whipping Cream, unwhipped
1/4 cup Splenda®, sugar substitute, divided
1/2 teaspoon Vanilla Extract
Dash Salt
Remaining Chocolate pudding mix from Cupcake recipe, (2 Tablespoons
    plus 1 teaspoon), page 143
1/2 cup Heavy Whipping Cream, whipped until thick
3 Tablespoons Water

In a small mixing bowl, whip cream cheese and butter until smooth and fluffy. Whip in unwhipped heavy whipping cream, Splenda®, vanilla extract, salt, and remaining chocolate pudding mix.

Fold whipped cream into chocolate mixture. Gradually stir in water 1 Tablespoon at a time to spreading consistency.

Frost cupcakes and store covered and refrigerated. Best served cold or frozen.

Note: This makes a generous amount of frosting for 18 cupcakes.

18 servings @ 1.5 grams of usable carbs each.

Chocolate Glaze

Servings: 6

1/2 square unsweetened Baking Chocolate
2 Tablespoons Butter, softened
1/4 cup Hot Water
1 1/2 teaspoons unsweetened Cocoa
1/4 cup Splenda®, sugar substitute
1/4 teaspoon Xanthan Gum
1/2 teaspoon liquid Sweet'N Low®, sugar substitute
1/4 teaspoon Vanilla Extract
2 Tablespoons Heavy Whipping Cream
Water to thin to glaze consistency

Melt baking chocolate and butter in a small microwave safe bowl 1-2 minutes on high, stirring every 30 seconds. Stir in hot water and set aside.

In a medium bowl whisk together cocoa, Splenda®, and Xanthan Gum. Whisk in chocolate and butter mixture, liquid Sweet'N Low®, vanilla extract, and heavy whipping cream. Whisk vigorously.

Thin with water if necessary to glaze consistency.

Note: Use on Boston Cream Pie, (page 136) or use as a delicious topping on any of your favorite desserts. Total recipe contains 9 grams of usable carbs.

6 servings @ 1.5 grams of usable carbs each.

Crust for Pies

1/4 cup Atkins® Bake Mix
1/2 teaspoon Guar Gum
2 Tablespoons Splenda®, sugar substitute
1/2 cup Heavy Whipping Cream
1 large Egg
1 teaspoon Vanilla Extract

Pre-heat oven to 350°

Whisk bake mix, Guar Gum, and Splenda® together in small mixing bowl. Whisk in heavy whipping cream, egg, and vanilla extract until smooth.

Let set for 10 minutes. Spread in 9" buttered pie pan. Bake @ 350° for

16-18 minutes or until set and browned around edges.

Cool in pan on rack.

Note: Great crust for Lemon Meringue Pie, (page 149).

Makes 1 recipe @ 9.8 grams of usable carbs total.

Variation:
Dessert Crust
1/4 cup Atkins® Bake Mix
1/2 teaspoon Guar Gum
2 Tablespoons Splenda®, sugar substitute
3/4 cup Heavy Whipping Cream
2 large Eggs
1 teaspoon Vanilla Extract

Pre-heat oven to 350°

Whisk first 3 ingredients together in medium bowl. Add remaining ingredients and whisk until fairly smooth. Pour into a sprayed 9"x13" cake pan and tap on countertop to level. Bake @ 350° for 15-20 minutes until beginning to lightly brown. Cool in pan on rack. For thicker crust, bake in 8" square or round pan. Will need extra time to bake.

Makes 1 recipe @ 13.6 grams of usable carbs total.

Sweetened Whipped Cream

Servings: 12

1 cup Heavy Whipping Cream
1/2 teaspoon Vanilla Extract
3 Tablespoons Splenda®, sugar substitute
1/8 teaspoon liquid Sweet'N Low®, sugar substitute

Whip ingredients together with an electric mixer until very thick. Do not over beat or it will turn to butter.

Refrigerate until serving time.

Note: Best served within 24 hours. Blend together just before serving and use on any of your favorite dessert recipes.

12 servings @ .9 grams of usable carbs each.

Variation:
Frozen Whipped Cream Clouds
Whip together Sweetened Whipped Cream ingredients until thick. Line an 11"x15" jelly roll pan with waxed paper or plastic wrap. Spoon whipped cream into 12 equal mounds, shaping nicely with spoon.

Make sure heavy whipping cream is whipped enough to hold its shape, but do not over whip or it will turn to butter. Place baking sheet in freezer until mounds are frozen solid. Then carefully remove them and place in a lock-top plastic bag. Store in freezer.

Use in Root Beer Float or Orange Dream recipes, (page 23) or place on any of your favorite desserts and let thaw.

12 servings @ .9 grams of usable carbs each.

Lemon Cheesecake

Servings: 16

5 - 8 ounce packages Cream Cheese, softened
1/4 pound Butter, softened (1 stick)
1 1/2 small boxes sugar-free Lemon Jell-O® (1/2 box = 1/2 Tablespoon
   plus a pinch)
1/3 cup Boiling Water
1/2 cup Heavy Whipping Cream
1 teaspoon grated Lemon Zest (just yellow part - no white)
2/3 cup Splenda®, sugar substitute
6 large Eggs, yolks broken

Pre-heat oven to 325°. Whip cream cheese and butter in a large bowl with an electric mixer until smooth and creamy. Dissolve Jell-O® in boiling water. Takes time to dissolve completely in small amount of water. Whip Jell-O® into cream cheese gradually. Add heavy whipping cream, Splenda®, and lemon zest and mix until blended. Add eggs and mix on low speed only until combined. DO NOT OVERMIX or texture will be grainy instead of creamy.

Pour into a 9" sprayed springform pan, I also line the bottom with parchment paper. Wrap outside bottom of pan and up sides with doubled aluminum foil to prevent leaking. Rap pan several times on countertop to release air bubbles.

Bake @ 325° for 60-70 minutes until just set. Turn oven off and leave in oven 1 additional hour. Finish cooling at room temperature. Do not remove sides of pan until completely cooled to room temperature. Cover and refrigerate at least 6 hours. Will get firmer as it chills.

Note: Top with your favorite Berry Sauce, (page 123) if desired. Be sure to count the extra carbs.

Variations:
Orange Cheesecake
Substitute equal amounts of Orange Zest and sugar-free Orange Jell-O®.

Lime Cheesecake
Substitute equal amounts of Lime Zest and sugar-free Lime Jell-O®.

16 servings @ 3.1 grams of usable carbs each.

Lemon Meringue Pie
Servings: 6

1 - recipe Crust for Pies, (page 146) prepare crust and set aside to cool

Filling:
1 cup Splenda®, sugar substitute
1/8 teaspoon Salt plus a pinch
1 1/2 teaspoons Xanthan Gum
1/2 teaspoon Guar Gum
1/2 cup fresh squeezed Lemon Juice
1 1/2 cups Cold Water
1 1/2 teaspoons Lemon Zest, grated (yellow part - no white)
3 large Egg yolks, slightly beaten
2 teaspoons liquid Sweet'N Low®, sugar substitute
1 1/2 Tablespoons Butter

Meringue:
1/4 cup Splenda®, sugar substitute
1 teaspoon Guar Gum
4 large Egg whites
1/2 teaspoon Cream of Tartar
1/2 teaspoon liquid Sweet'N Low®, sugar substitute
1/4 teaspoon Vanilla Extract

Filling:
Mix Splenda®, salt, Xanthan Gum, and Guar Gum in a medium heavy saucepan. Whisk in lemon juice and water. Cook over medium heat stirring constantly until just beginning to boil. Briskly whisk 2 Tablespoons lemon mixture into egg yolks. Then whisk in another 2 Tablespoons. Slowly pour yolk mixture into pan, whisking briskly. Reduce heat and continue to cook over low heat another 10 minutes, stirring frequently. Stir in lemon zest, butter and liquid Sweet'N Low®. Pour into cooled pie crust.

Meringue:
Pre-heat oven to 400°

Mix Splenda® and Guar Gum in a small bowl and set aside. Whip egg whites and cream of tartar in a medium mixing bowl with an electric mixer until soft peak stage. While mixer is running add liquid Sweet'N Low® and vanilla extract. Continue whipping while adding Splenda® mixture 1 Tablespoon at a time. Whip until very stiff. Spread over lemon filling. Make sure to seal to crust. Bake for about 10 minutes.

6 servings @ 8.6 grams of usable carbs each.

Lime Frosted Jell-O

Servings: 10

2 small packages sugar-free Lime Jell-O®, divided (remove 1/2 teaspoon
     and set aside)
1 Tablespoon Boiling Water
1 cup Heavy Whipping Cream
1 Tablespoon sugar-free Jell-O® instant Vanilla pudding mix
1 teaspoon Lime Zest, grated (green part - no white)

Make Jell-O® with 1 3/4 cups boiling water in an oblong glass dish. Stir well until dissolved then add 2 cups cold water and refrigerate until set. Dissolve 1/2 teaspoon of reserved Jell-O® in 1 Tablespoon boiling water, set aside to cool at room temperature.

Whip remaining ingredients together, including cooled 1/2 teaspoon

Jell-O®, in a medium mixing bowl with an electric mixer until thick.

Spread over set Jell-O® and chill. At serving time cut into 10 equal servings.

10 servings @ 1.1 grams of usable carbs each.

Old-Fashioned Vanilla Pudding

Servings: 3

1 cup Heavy Whipping Cream
1/2 cup Water
3 large Egg yolks
1/4 cup Splenda®, sugar substitute
1 teaspoon Xanthan Gum
1/2 teaspoon Vanilla Extract
1/4 teaspoon Almond Extract
1/2 teaspoon liquid Sweet'N Low®, sugar substitute

Heat cream and water in a medium, heavy saucepan until hot but not boiling. Skin will form on top. While cream and water are heating, beat egg yolks with a fork in a small bowl just until smooth. Set aside. Mix Splenda® and Xanthan Gum in a separate small bowl and set aside. When cream is hot, add a small amount very slowly, about 2-3 Tablespoons to egg yolks, stirring quickly with a fork. Add another 2-3 Tablespoons hot cream very slowly to egg yolks, stirring quickly with a fork. Pour yolk mixture slowly into remaining cream in saucepan whisking briskly. Reduce heat to low and sprinkle Splenda® mixture gradually over pudding and whisk in until smooth. Cook for 3-4 minutes until thickened, then remove from heat. Add extracts and pour into a plastic bowl.

Note: If mixture separates, let cool a bit and whisk until creamy. Cover with plastic wrap directly on pudding so skin won't form. Whisk in liquid Sweet'N Low® after pudding has cooled. Refrigerate covered.

Note: Fabulous filling for Boston Creme Pie, (page 136).

3 - 1/2 cup servings @ 4.4 grams of usable carbs each.

Variation:
Chocolate Pudding
Add 2 Tablespoons of unsweetened Cocoa with the Splenda® mixture and omit the Almond Extract.

3 - 1/2 cup servings @ 5.1 grams of usable carbs each.

Peanut Butter & Chocolate Patties

Servings: 32

4 ounces Cream Cheese, softened
1/4 pound Butter, softened (1 stick)
1/2 cup smooth Peanut Butter or low carb Peanut Butter (no more than 6 grams of carbs per 2 Tablespoons)
5 Tablespoons Splenda®, sugar substitute
1/2 teaspoon liquid Sweet'N Low®, sugar substitute
1 teaspoon Vanilla Extract

Whip cream cheese in a medium bowl with an electric mixer until smooth. Add remaining ingredients and whip until smooth. Spread evenly in an 8" square pan lined with waxed paper. Refrigerate until firm.

Coating:

4 Tablespoons skinless, salted Peanuts, chopped very fine (food processor works best)
3 Tablespoons unsweetened Cocoa
6 Tablespoons Splenda®, sugar substitute
1 Tablespoons sugar-free Jell-O® instant Chocolate pudding mix

Mix all ingredients in a small bowl. Set aside.

Turn out candy onto a cutting board and peel off waxed paper. Divide into 32 equal pieces. Shape into patties and roll in coating.

Refrigerate covered or freeze.

32 servings @ 1.4 grams of usable carbs.

Pistachio Ice Cream

Servings: 12

2 1/2 cups Heavy Whipping Cream
1/2 cup Water
1/2 cup natural Pistachio Nuts, shelled and chopped
1/2 cup Splenda®, sugar substitute
2 teaspoons liquid Sweet'N Low®, sugar substitute
1 teaspoon Almond Extract
8 drops Green Food Coloring (optional)

Whisk all ingredients together in a medium bowl until well blended. Pour into freezer bowl of ice cream maker while running and run for about 25 minutes or until thick.

Pour into paper cups, 1/2 cup into each, and freeze covered with plastic wrap.

You can thaw each serving on low in the microwave for 15 seconds.

Note: If you don't have an ice cream maker, after whisking all ingredients together, freeze in bowl until starting to get thick. Whip with an electric mixer, then pour into cups and cover with plastic wrap. Freeze.

12 servings @ 4.1 grams of usable carbs each.

Pumpkin Pecan Dessert
Servings: 8

3/4 cup Splenda®, sugar substitute
2 1/4 teaspoons Ground Cinnamon, divided
3/4 teaspoon Ground Ginger
1/4 teaspoon Ground Cloves
1/2 teaspoon Salt
1 - 16 ounce can 100% pure Pumpkin (do not use Pumpkin Pie mix)
1 cup Heavy Whipping Cream
1/4 cup Sour Cream
3 large Eggs, slightly beaten
1 Tablespoon Brown Sugar Twin®, sugar substitute
3 Tablespoons toasted Pecans, chopped small

Pre-heat oven to 325°

Whisk together Splenda®, 2 teaspoons ground cinnamon, ginger, cloves, salt, pumpkin, heavy whipping cream, sour cream, and eggs in a medium mixing bowl until well blended.

Pour evenly into 8 sprayed custard cups. Sprinkle tops with Brown Sugar Twin® and remaining ground cinnamon then pecans.

Bake @ 325° for 30-40 minutes or until center is almost set. Cool on a rack. Cover and chill until cold.

Note: I use Libby's® brand Pumpkin. Also delicious topped with Sweetened Whipped Cream, (page 147) but be sure to count the extra carbs.

8 servings @ 6 grams of usable carbs each.

Strawberry Cheesecake

Servings: 16

5 - 8 ounce packages Cream Cheese, softened
1/4 pound Butter, softened (1 stick)
1 1/2 small boxes, sugar-free Strawberry Jell-O®
(1/2 box = 1/2 Tablespoon plus a pinch)
1/3 cup Boiling Water
1/2 cup Heavy Whipping Cream
1 cup Strawberries, chopped
3/4 cup Splenda®, sugar substitute
6 large Eggs, yolks broken

Pre-heat oven to 325°

Whip cream cheese and butter in a large bowl with an electric mixer until smooth and creamy. Set aside. Dissolve Jell-O® in boiling water. Takes time to dissolve completely in small amount of water.

Whip Jell-O® into cream cheese gradually. Add heavy whipping cream, Splenda®, and strawberries and whip until well mixed. Add eggs and mix on low speed only until combined. DO NOT OVERMIX or texture will be grainy instead of creamy.

Spray a 9" springform pan, I also line bottom with parchment paper, and wrap outside bottom and up sides with doubled aluminum foil to prevent leakage. Pour mixture into pan and rap several times on countertop to release air bubbles.

Bake @ 325° for 60-70 minutes until just set. Turn off oven and leave in 1 additional hour. Finish cooling at room temperature. Do not remove sides of pan until completely cooled to room temperature. Cover and refrigerate at least 6 hours before serving. Will get firmer as it chills.

Note: Great topped with Strawberry Sauce, (page 123) and/or Sweetened Whipped Cream, (page 147). Just remember to count the extra carbs.

16 servings @ 3.8 grams of usable carbs each.

Strawberry Crepes
Servings: 6

3 large Eggs
2/3 cup Heavy Whipping Cream
3 Tablespoons Atkins® Bake Mix
4 Tablespoons Splenda®, sugar substitute
1/8 teaspoon Almond Extract
1/4 teaspoon Vanilla Extract
1/2 teaspoon grated Orange Zest (Orange part only)
Butter (use amount necessary to fry Crepes)

Strawberry Filling:
2 cups Strawberries, washed, hulled, and sliced (reserve a few slices for garnish)
6 Tablespoons Splenda®, sugar substitute
1 - recipe Sweetened Whipped Cream, (page 147)

Whisk together all crepe ingredients in a medium bowl. Melt about 1 Tablespoon of butter in a heavy 8" skillet or crepe pan over medium heat.

When foam subsides, pour 1/6 of batter in pan and tilt pan to cover entire bottom evenly. Cook until lightly browned on underside and top side is set. Turn carefully and cook until other side starts to brown. Remove from pan and place between paper towels.

Repeat with remaining batter. This can be done ahead, just wrap with plastic wrap after they have cooled until serving time.

Strawberry Filling:
Combine strawberries and Splenda® and place 1/4 cup on each Crepe and roll up. Place each on dessert plate. Spoon sweetened whipped cream over each Crepe and garnish with rest of strawberries.

Note: This makes a wonderful breakfast or light dessert.

6 servings @ 8.3 grams of usable carbs each.

Strawberry-Kiwi Puff

Servings: 12

2 small boxes, sugar-free Strawberry-Kiwi Jell-O®, prepared as directed
1 1/2 cups Heavy Whipping Cream
1/2 teaspoon Vanilla Extract
3 Tablespoons Splenda®, sugar substitute, divided
1 teaspoon sugar-free Strawberry Jell-O®, dry
1 1/2 cups sliced Strawberries, mixed with 1 Tablespoon Splenda®, sugar
   substitute

Pour prepared strawberry-kiwi Jell-O® into 8"x11.5" rectangular glass dish. Refrigerate until set.

Whip heavy whipping cream, vanilla extract, remaining 2 Tablespoons Splenda®, and dry Jell-O® until very thick soft peaks. Stir in strawberries and spread evenly over Jell-O®, then chill. When ready to serve cut into 12 equal servings.

12 servings @ 2.1 grams of usable carbs each.

Strawberry Snowballs
Servings: 8

Base Layer:
Butter for greasing muffin cups
2 large Eggs
1 cup Heavy Whipping Cream
1/2 cup Water
1 Tablespoon sugar-free Jell-O® instant Vanilla pudding mix
1 teaspoon Vanilla Extract
1/4 teaspoon Almond Extract
1 Tablespoon Atkins® Bake Mix
1 Tablespoon Splenda®, sugar substitute
1/2 teaspoon Guar Gum

Strawberry Layer:
1 cup Strawberries, washed, hulled, and sliced
1/2 teaspoon liquid Sweet'N Low®, sugar substitute

Topping:
1 1/2 cups Heavy Whipping Cream
1 1/2 teaspoons Vanilla Extract
4 Tablespoons Splenda®, sugar substitute

Pre-heat oven to 325°

Base Layer: Butter 8 standard non-stick muffin cups. Half fill any empty ones with water to prevent pan from warping. In a medium bowl whisk eggs, heavy whipping cream, and water until well combined. Add remaining ingredients and whisk until nearly smooth. Pour into prepared pans, dividing evenly. Bake @ 325° for 30 minutes or until set and slightly browned. Cool on rack. When cool, place each in a dessert dish and refrigerate until cold.

Strawberry Layer: In small bowl, combine strawberries and liquid Sweet'N Low®. Top each base with strawberry layer, dividing equally.

Topping: Whip all ingredients until very thick. Spread topping over strawberries and refrigerate until serving time.

8 servings @ 4.7 grams of usable carbs each.

INDEX

Appetizers & Snacks

BBQ Meatballs 10
Deep Fried Cajun Cauliflower 11
Deli Meat Rolls 12
French Deviled Eggs 13
Guacamole 14
Ham & Spinach Drops 15
Sauerkraut & Ham Balls 16
Rueben Balls 16
Sausage Stuffed Mushroom Caps
with Pesto Cream Sauce 17
Savory Stuffed Mushrooms 18
Smoked Sausage Appetizers 19
Teriyaki Chicken Wings 20

Beverages

Chocolate Shake 22
Strawberry Shake 22
Tutti Frutti Shake 22
Root Beer Float 23
Orange Dream 23
Hot Chocolate 24
Mexican Hot Chocolate 24

Breads

Butterscotch Pecan Muffins 26
Garlic Poppyseed Rolls 27
Ham & Cheese Breakfast Muffins 28
Hush Puppies 29
Sour Cream Poppyseed Muffins 30
Spice Doughnut Holes 31
Strawberry Walnut Muffins 32

Breakfasts

Cauliflower & Ham Quiche 34
Crustless Asparagus & Ham Quiche 35
Ham Hash & Eggs 36
Italian Frittata 37
Pancakes with Maple Syrup 38
Pork Carnitas Frittata 39
Puffy Baked Eggs 40
Quick & Easy Tex-Mex Eggs 41
Salsa Scramble 42
Swiss Eggs & Sausage 43
Taco Omelets 44

Soups

Chili 46
Cream of Broccoli Soup 47
Ham & Asparagus Soup 48
Oyster Stew 49
Turkey Egg Drop Soup 50

Salads & Salad Dressings

Cabbage & Bacon Salad 52
Confetti Salad 53
Creamy Cole Slaw 54
Dilled Creamed Cucumbers 55
Grilled Chicken Salad
with Vegetables 56
Pork Salad 57
Roast Beef Salad 58
Sweet Cauliflower with Bacon Salad 59
Taco Salad 60
Turkey Salad 61
Mediterranean Chicken Salad 62
Bleu Cheese Dressing 63
Ranch Dressing 64
Red French Dressing 65
Sun-Dried Tomato Mushroom
Vinaigrette Dressing 66
Sweet Mayonnaise for
Miracle Whip Lovers 67
Thousand Island Dressing 68

Entrees

BEEF

Chicken Fried Steak 70
Ground Beef & Cabbage Casserole 71
Hamburger Mushroom &
Green Bean Casserole 72
Baked Italian Deli Sandwich 73
Meatballs Alfredo 74
Mexi Stuffed Peppers 75
Mexican Pizza 76
Mexican Pizza Crust 77
Old-Fashioned Meatloaf 78
Pizza Roll Meatloaf 79
Prime Rib with Mushroom Au Jus 80
Quick Chow Mein 81

EAT YOURSELF THIN LIKE I DID!

Rueben Lasagna 82
Taco Meat 83

PORK
Quick Hot Deli Plate 84
BBQ Ribs 85
Fresh Pork with Sauerkraut
Cabbage & Tomatoes 86
Fried Smoked Sausage 87
Ham Patties 88
Pizza 89
Pizza Crust 90
Pork & Cabbage with Sauerkraut 91
Pork Chops with Cream Gravy 92
Sweet & Sour Pork 99
Sweet & Sour Pork Vegetable Stir Fry 93
Zucchini Boats 94

POULTRY
Chicken Cacciatore 95
Chicken Olé 96
Chicken Parmigiana 97
Quick Swiss Chicken with Broccoli 98
Sweet & Sour Chicken 99

FISH & SEAFOOD
Broiled Halibut
with Citrus Dill Butter 100
Crispy Fried Fish 101
Crusty Cajun Salmon
with Cajun Mayonnaise 102
Greek Baked Salmon 103
Salmon Patties 104
Shrimp Scampi Parmesano 105
Sweet & Sour Shrimp 99

Vegetables
Baked "Potato" Casserole 107
Cauliflower Scramble 108
Creole Green Beans 109
Eggplant Parmigiana 110
Grilled Portobello Mushroom Caps 111
Ham & Swiss Green Beans 112
Italian Spinach 113
Marvelous Mushrooms 114
"Potato" Latke Pancakes 115
Sautéed Sesame Asparagus 116
Sweet & Spicy Red Cabbage 117
Zucchini Alfredo 118
Zucchini Italian Style 119

Sauce & Condiments
Alfredo Sauce 121
BBQ Sauce 122
Berry Sauce 123
Marinara Sauce 124
Nancy's Ketchup 125
Nancy's Pico de Gallo 126
Nancy's Steak Sauce 127
Nancy's Strawberry Spread 128
Nancy's Maple Butter 128
Nancy's Vanilla Butter 128
Pesto Cream Sauce 129
Spicy Seafood Cocktail Sauce 130
Sweet & Sour Sauce 131
Sweet Zesty Mustard Sauce 132
Nancy's Tartar Sauce 133

Desserts
Blueberry Dream Squares 135
Boston Crème Pie 136
Butterscotch Pecan Cheesecake 137
Cherry Cinnamon Dessert 138
Cherry Swirl 139
Chinese Almond Cookies 140
Chocolate Almond Ice Cream 141
Chocolate Cheesecake 142
Chocolate Cupcakes 143
Chocolate Cream Frosting 144
Chocolate Glaze 145
Crust for Pie 146
Dessert Crust 146
Frozen Whipped Cream Clouds 147
Lemon Cheesecake 148
Orange Cheesecake 148
Lime Cheesecake 148
Lemon Meringue Pie 149
Lime Frosted Jell-O 150
Old-Fashioned Vanilla Pudding 151
Chocolate Pudding 151
Peanut Butter & Chocolate Patties 152
Pistachio Ice Cream 153
Pumpkin Pecan Dessert 154
Strawberry Cheesecake 155
Strawberry Crepes 156
Strawberry-Kiwi Puff 157
Strawberry Snowballs 158
Sweetened Whipped Cream 147

EAT YOURSELF THIN LIKE I DID!